AF593602

THELMA BROWN'S SILHOUETTE BOOK OF SLIMMING

THELMA BROWN'S

SILHOUETTE
BOOK OF SLIMMING

Zita Alden

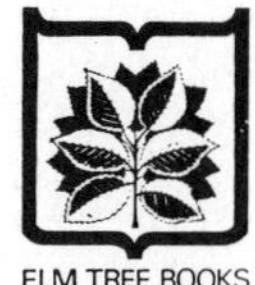

ELM TREE BOOKS · HAMISH HAMILTON · LONDON

First published in Great Britain 1972
by Elm Tree Books Limited
90 Great Russell Street London WC1

SBN 241 02164 2

Design and illustrations by
Norma Crockford

Printed Photolitho in Great Britain by
Ebenezer Baylis and Son Ltd.
The Trinity Press
Worcester, and London

CONTENTS

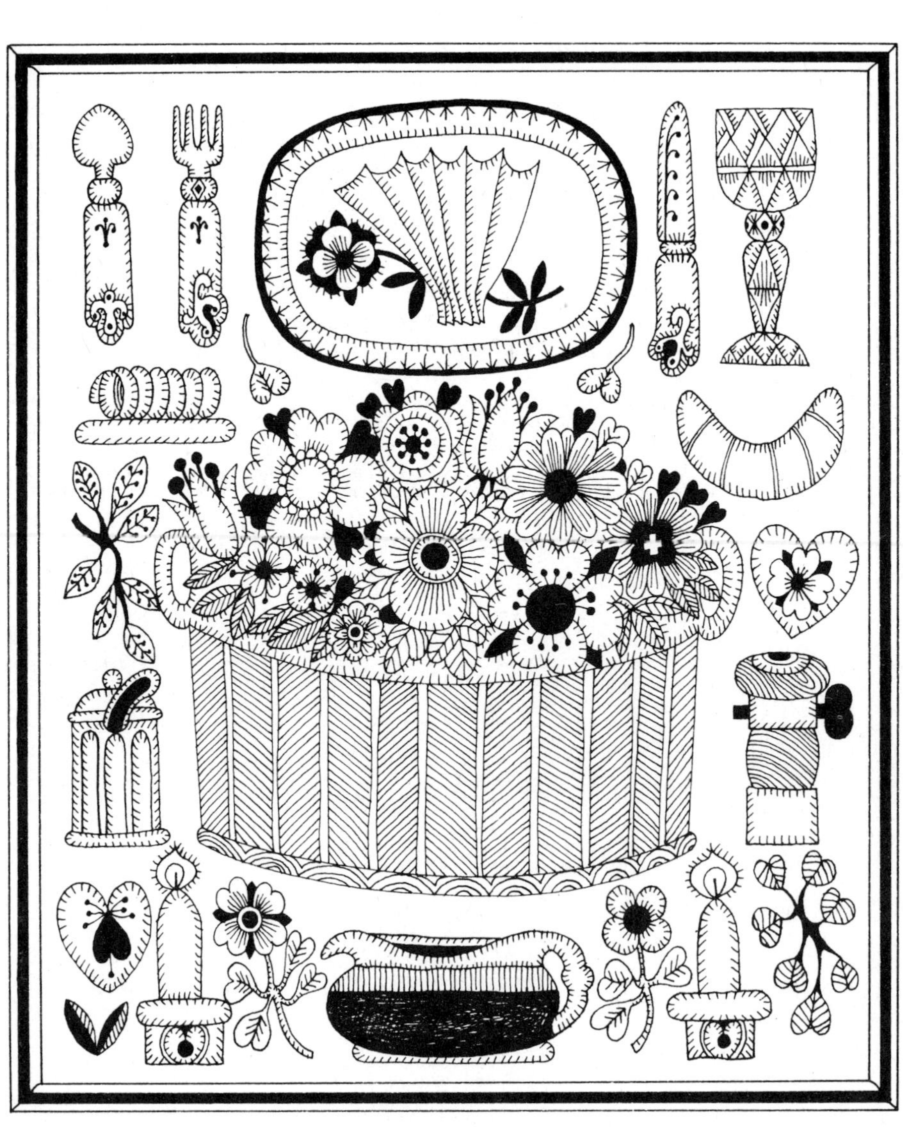

ACKNOWLEDGEMENTS

The author would like to thank Dorothy Parkes for her research assistance, Sarah Hodge, the home economist who checked the recipes, Carolyn Saunders, dietitian, and the following for recipes and pictorial help:

Angel Studios
Australian Recipe Service
Baco Foil
Bird's Eye Foods Ltd
Blue Band Margarine
British Egg Information Service
British Sugar Bureau
Butter Information Council
Canned and Packaged Foods Bureau
Cheese Bureau
Delrosa
Eden Vale
Food Information Centre
Flour Advisory Bureau
Fruit Producers' Council
Gale's Honey
Guernsey Tomato Board
General Electric Co
H. J. Heinz & Co Ltd
Justina Wine Co
Kraft Margarine
Malayan Pineapple Board
Nestlé Co Ltd
Oxo Potato Marketing Board
Rowntrees Jelly
Walls Sausages
Walls Ice Cream

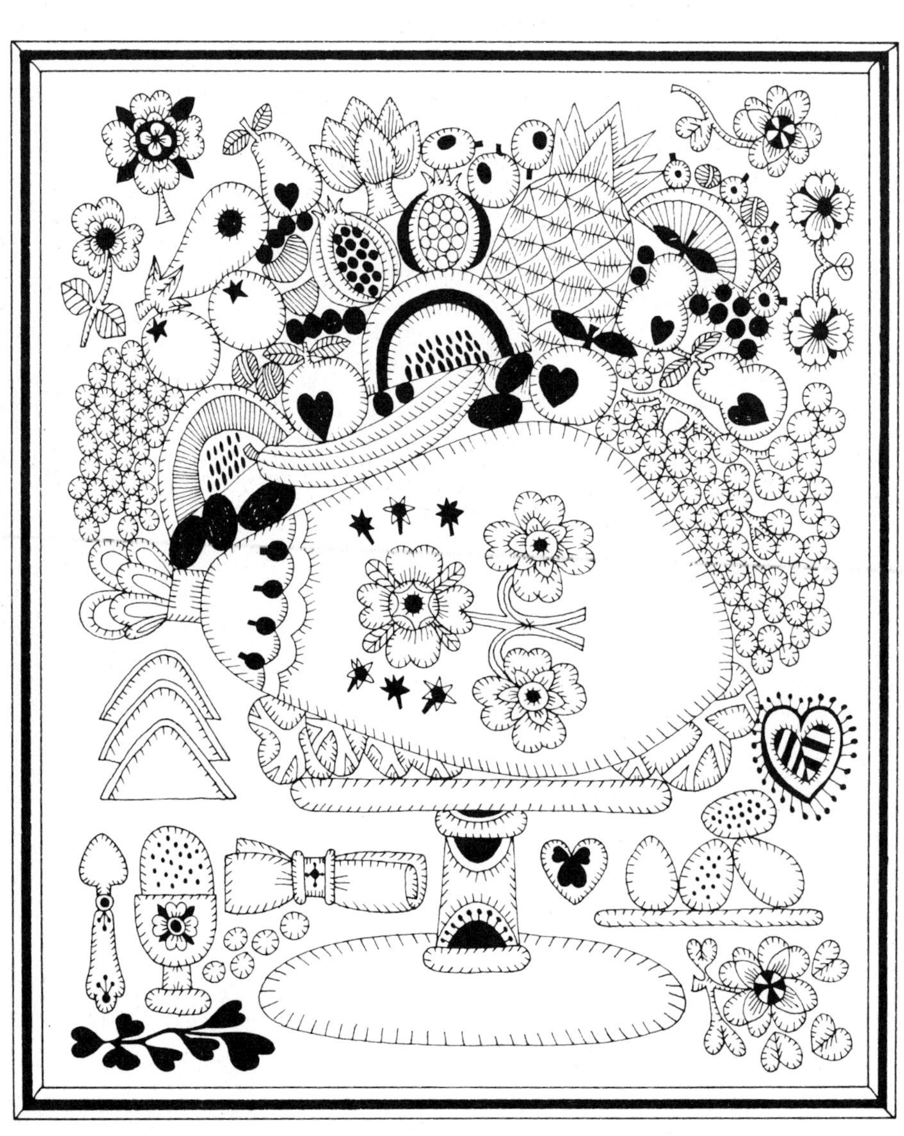

FOREWORD

I am sure that this cookery book will strike you as being very unusual. It is a slimming cookery book that advocates the *full* enjoyment of *all* foods, not just a limited selection. I myself have always enjoyed eating good food and now, with the Silhouette Slimming Club method of dieting. I am able to live my life to the full without depriving myself of the foods I love.

When I was very overweight the stumbling block with every diet I tried was the forbidden food list. If it banned chocolate I craved for chocolate, if it disallowed cakes and sugar I began to fancy meringues. Then I invented my points system, ate everything I liked with one eye on my points table, lost weight and really enjoyed life for the first time in fifteen years.

Thus I had proved that the quantity is more damaging then the quality.

With our suggested 'basic allowance' for health and the points method which every individual with any tastes can adapt, you too can EAT AND GET SLIM.

THELMA BROWN

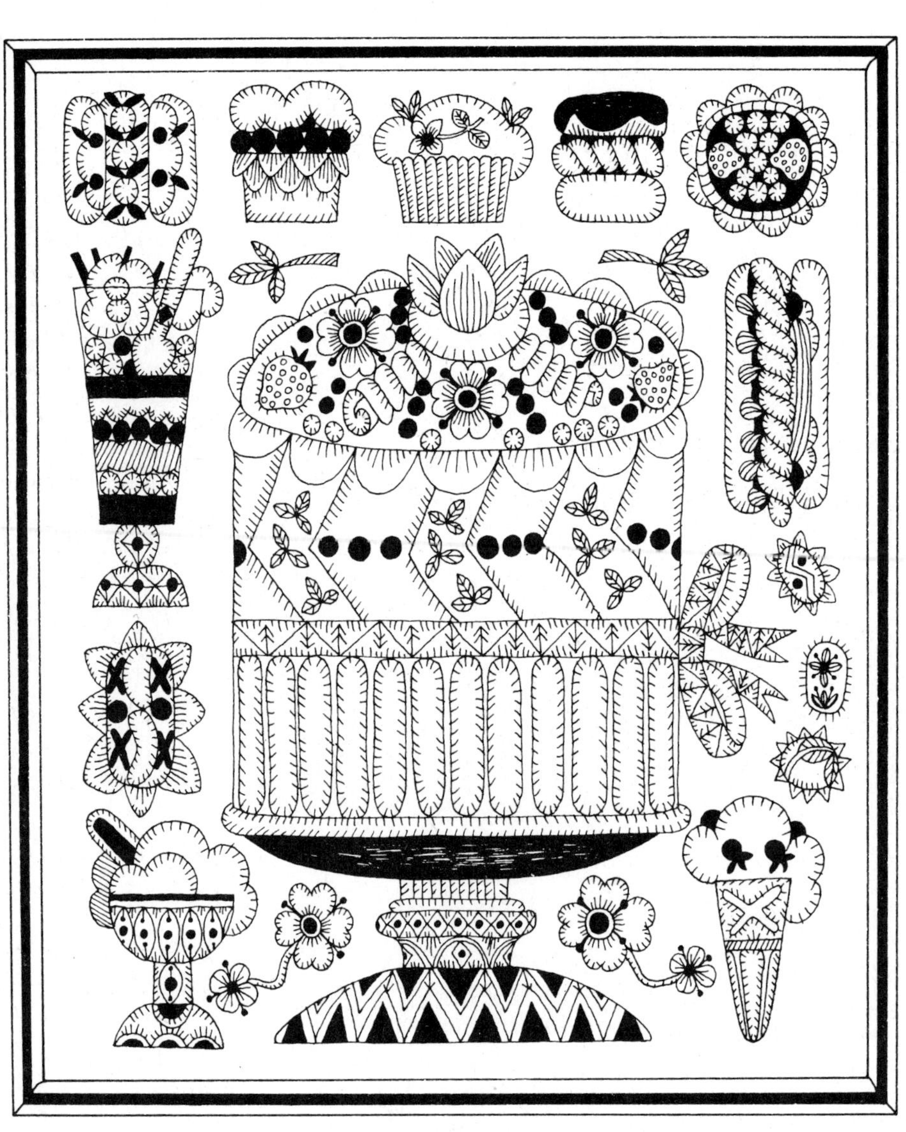

HOW SILHOUETTE BEGAN

This cookery book is dedicated, like myself and the Silhouette Slimming Club, to fat people, especially the thousands of fat people who enjoy good food yet wish to be slim. All those words – stout, plump, solid, chubby, puppy fat, obese, overweight, heavy – are kinder ways of avoiding the reality of being F-A-T. Every time I see a fat person my heart goes out to them. Having been overweight myself for fifteen long and miserable years I know the terrible feeling of having tried everything and failed totally.

I used every excuse in the book, and invented a few more besides, to explain to myself why I was fat. One thing more than any other kept dragging me back above the thirteen stone mark – forbidden food. It did not matter what food my diet banned, within hours I developed a craving for it. Especially my great love – chocolate.

I do not just eat to live, I honestly live to eat. Most fat people are the same. I know with me it was always far too long before the next meal. Before I started lunch, I was planning tea and then dinner. I always ate chocolate as though someone were about to snatch the box away from me. And then I would feel guilty and miserable, which meant I would head for the cake tin or the bread box. Fat people are made to feel guilty about their eating, but why should we give it up any more than giving up other pleasures such as drinking, talking, sex or even smoking? The secret, of course, is that magic word 'moderation'. Apply this to the enjoyable things of life and they become even more pleasurable and this forms the basis of the tremendous success that Silhouette Slimming Club has experienced.

It took me fifteen long years to realize that I enjoyed eating so much that I was prepared to suffer agonies mentally and, to a certain extent, physically, rather than live only on the foods suggested in so many diets, leaving alone that lovely list of forbidden foods. I tried every trick to get slim: pills, potions, faddy foods, bribes and bets, even religion.
I tried everything until the wonderful day – I didn't realize it at the time – that I accepted the fact that, pig though I might sound, I would slim only by eating

everything — by disciplining myself on quantities. I had, by this time, read a lot of books on nutrition, and realized that you are what you eat. So I tried with 1,250 calories a day first of all, but found being only human I would often cheat a little here and there and the result was too many calories. I cut the allowance to 1,000 and this gave a more satisfactory result. I gave myself a basic allowance of what I knew to be health-giving foods, then took great delight in adding some of my favourite foods — chocolate, rice pudding, fresh cream cakes. But not all in one day.

Having organized the most delightful part, I felt a little help was needed and asked a girl I knew slightly through my husband's business (friends are no good for this) to try my diet recipe. We weighed ourselves and kept in contact by telephone. A miracle happened — it began to work — it took months (not weeks) but the joy of seeing the scales creeping down instead of up is something only a fat person can experience.

This led to the Silhouette Slimming Club as it stands today. Hundreds of classes all over Britain, in villages and cities, hamlets and towns — wherever there are sufficient fat ladies to form a class, Silhouette is there to help. We are unique in that we recognize that you need to be able to eat to your own preferences at times and that everyone is an individual with personal tastes. You can eat and get slim as the personal histories on pages 13–15 show. Every one of those people had given up hope of losing weight until they found Silhouette.

But do not expect the classes to do it all. You must really want to lose weight yourself. To support our group slimming classes I introduced voluntary isometric exercises. These are simply muscle contractions which are totally different from the normal 'keep fit' gymnastics. They are very easy to do and are marvellous at reducing inches in the strategic parts to complement the weight you are losing.

If you want us to help you, contact your nearest Silhouette area manager (see the list at the back of this book). We look forward to seeing you.

SILHOUETTE SUCCESS STORIES

I have been overweight since I was nine or ten. I like all fattening things like bread, pudding, fish and chips, cakes. Eight months before my twenty-first birthday I joined Silhouette Slimming Club, determined to lose five stone. The photographs *(below)* show the difference it made.

The things I like best about losing weight are being able to buy modern clothes without having to try on everything in the shop before finding something to fit me. I also find clothes in smaller sizes are much cheaper and can buy two dresses for the price of one.

My measurements now are 38–30–40 (dress size 16) much different from my former 49–45–56 (dress size 24).

The girls at work say that I look a lot better for losing weight and I think I am more lively and active. I enjoy going out of an evening and I don't mind going shopping and walking around the town. There was a time when I could not walk a hundred yards without being out of breath and my legs aching.

I find I take more interest in my appearance when I go out and I feel much healthier. I don't feel so old-fashioned now that I am able to wear more up-to-date clothes.

Before joining Silhouette I did try other diets but I like the atmosphere of Silhouette. I feel the Club's diet has given me confidence to do many things I would not have done before.

Valerie Sullivan
Brentwood, Essex

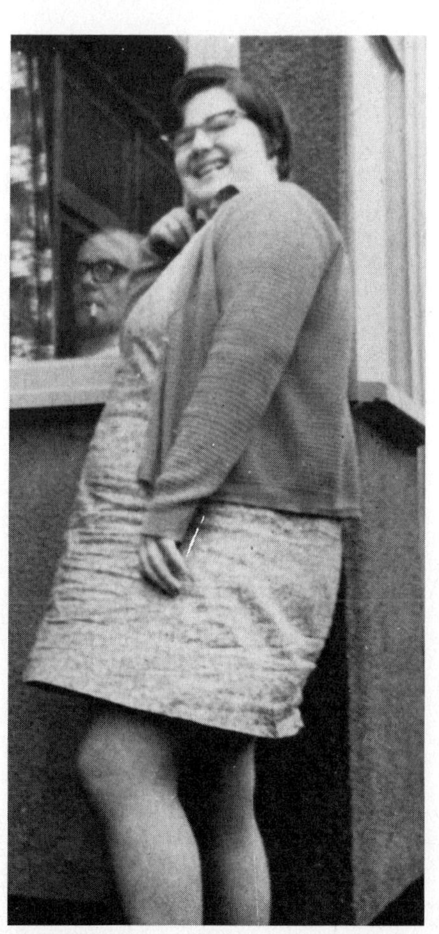

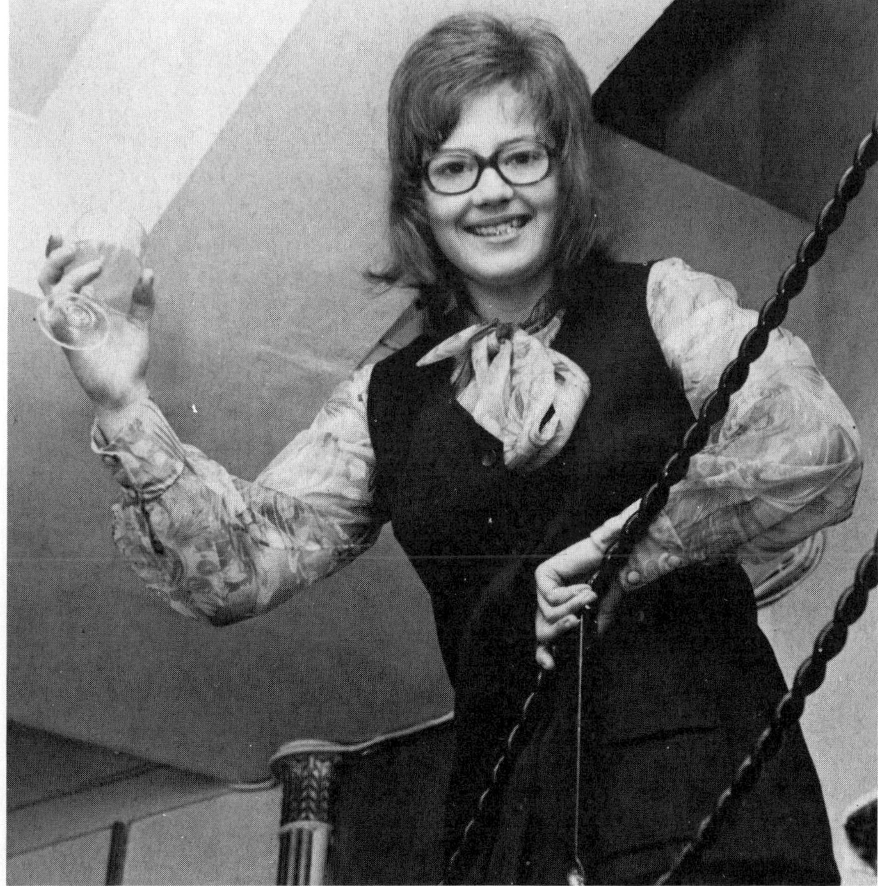

In all I've lost 7 stone 4 pounds and now weigh 9 stone 13 pounds.

I was an 11-pound baby and carried on from there. At the age of 14 I weighed well over 16 stone and because of my weight I had no enjoyable teenage years: no swimming, dancing or boy-friends. I was very unhappy, felt terribly self-conscious and the more unhappy I got the more I ate.

After leaving school I went to various doctors to see if they could help. I was given the usual tablets and lost weight but I eventually became addicted to the drugs and took them for the lift they gave me. They no longer took hunger away. I began to put all the weight on again. I then went to a Harley Street specialist, but that didn't really work. I tried various other methods, including hypnosis, without success. I then resigned myself to being fat until I joined Silhouette.

My husband married me while I was fat — for love — not looks. He has always been wonderful about my weight and helped if he could. He is now delighted with his 'new' wife.

The children are also delighted. I no longer get asked, 'Why are you fat, Mummy?' or told, 'My friend said you are fat.' My eldest daughter is only too keen to borrow my clothes and, at size 12 I can even wear hers.

It has made a terrific difference to my life, I have doors opened for me; men drivers give way on the roads, all the little things that never happened before. And the weight is staying off.

Rosalie Johns
Guildford, Surrey

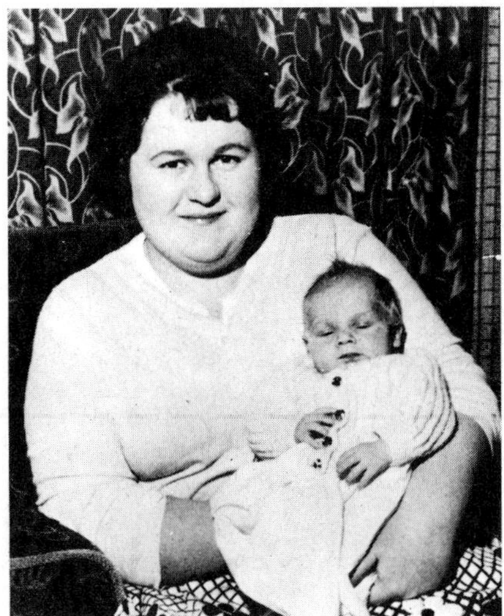

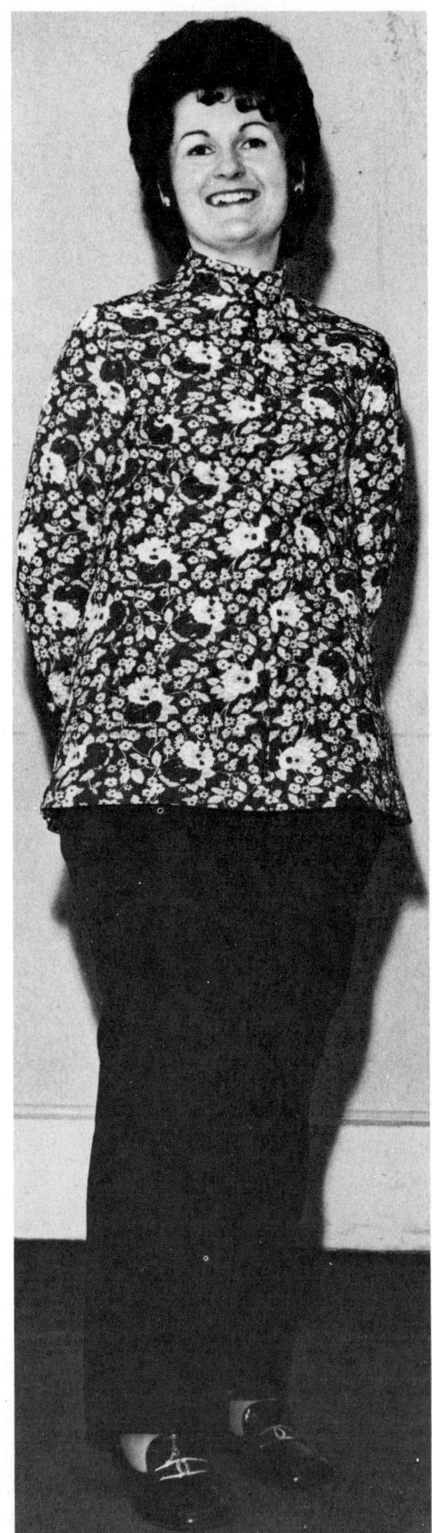

I was overweight from about the age of 8, always the fattest girl in the class. During my late teens I did manage to slim down a little, and when I was married at the age of 20, I was about 12 stone. From then on things changed; each year saw me a stone or more heavier and a few sizes larger, until I reached the grand total of 18 stone 9 pounds with a 53-inch hip measurement. I really think this would have carried on indefinitely if I hadn't met Thelma Brown and Silhouette.

After my first meeting with Thelma I returned home with a lot of hope but not a great deal of confidence as I had tried so many times to slim. After the first four or five weeks with a loss of nearly two stone I became dedicated to Thelma's methods.

Twelve months later, with a much slimmer me (and a changing personality), my husband decided he'd better have a go at slimming. At that time he weighed nearly 19 stone, had a 48-inch chest, a 50-inch waist and an awful problem with clothes. Now he's down to 13 stone with a 42-inch chest and a 38-inch waist, and much more vitality. People we haven't seen for a couple of years don't recognize us now.

It has really changed our lives. Before we lost the weight we had got to the stage when we just didn't go out. Now we take every opportunity of going out and even if we are the only couple on the dance floor neither of us minds. We take our two children swimming (they'd never even been to the baths). We've spent holidays wearing bathing suits on the beach. A couple of years ago I couldn't even have bought a bathing suit let alone have worn it.

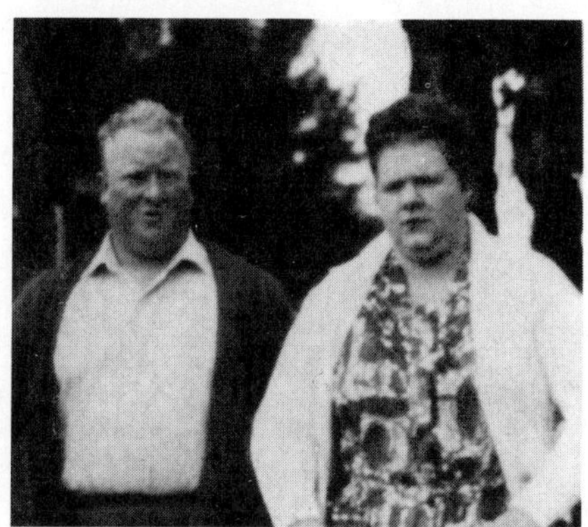

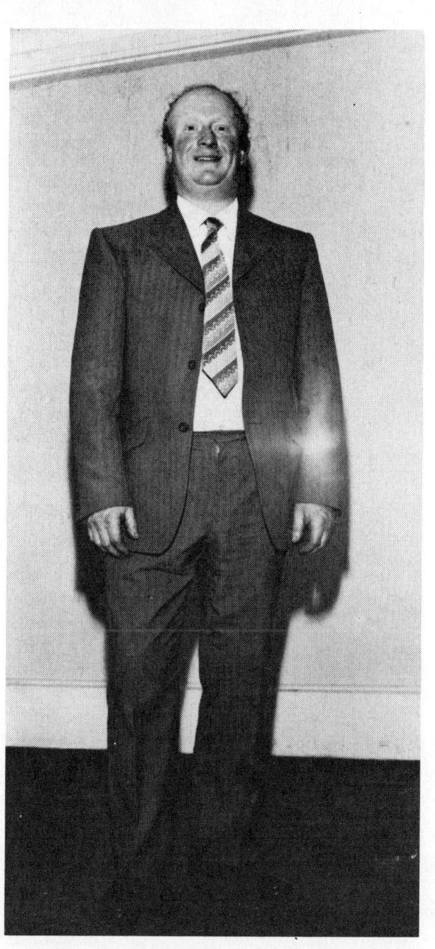

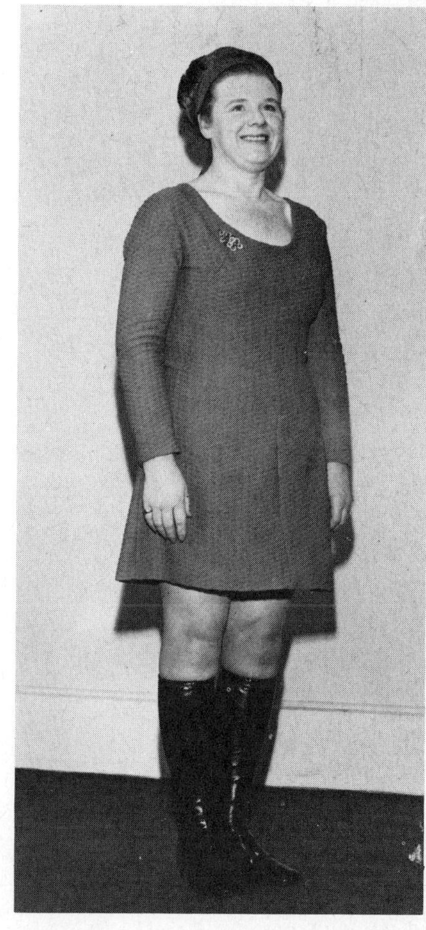

We still like and eat most things although our eating habits are different. We really do enjoy everything that we eat.

Vilma Haslehurst
Cudworth, Near Barnsley
Yorkshire

THE SILHOUETTE SECRET

Medically approved, Silhouette slimming is based on a points system in which 1 point is equal to 25 calories. You are allowed up to 40 points a day on a weekly basis so that if you are going to a wedding you can save 2 or 3 daily points from the preceding Sunday to Friday to use up in a spree at the Saturday festivities.

Every recipe in this book has a points value indicated by a large numeral, i.e.

10

---

and there is a list on pages 102–106 giving the points values of the main recipe ingredients.

The points value covers the whole recipe and should be divided by the number of servings to obtain the points value per person.

GUIDE TO WEIGHTS AND MEASURES

LEVEL SPOON MEASURES

1 tablespoon	=	2 dessertspoons
1 dessertspoon	=	2 teaspoons

LIQUID MEASURES

$\frac{1}{4}$ pint	=	5 fluid ounces
$\frac{1}{2}$ pint	=	10 fluid ounces
1 pint	=	20 fluid ounces

EACH OF THE FOLLOWING WEIGH APPROXIMATELY ONE OUNCE:

Level tablespoons

2	Flour, cornflour (similar ingredients)
5	fresh breadcrumbs
1	Rice, raw
2	Rice, boiled
1	Sugar, white or brown
1	Jam, honey, syrup or treacle
2	Sultanas or raisins
2	Nuts, shelled
2	Cooking or salad oil

Egg and Cheese Dishes

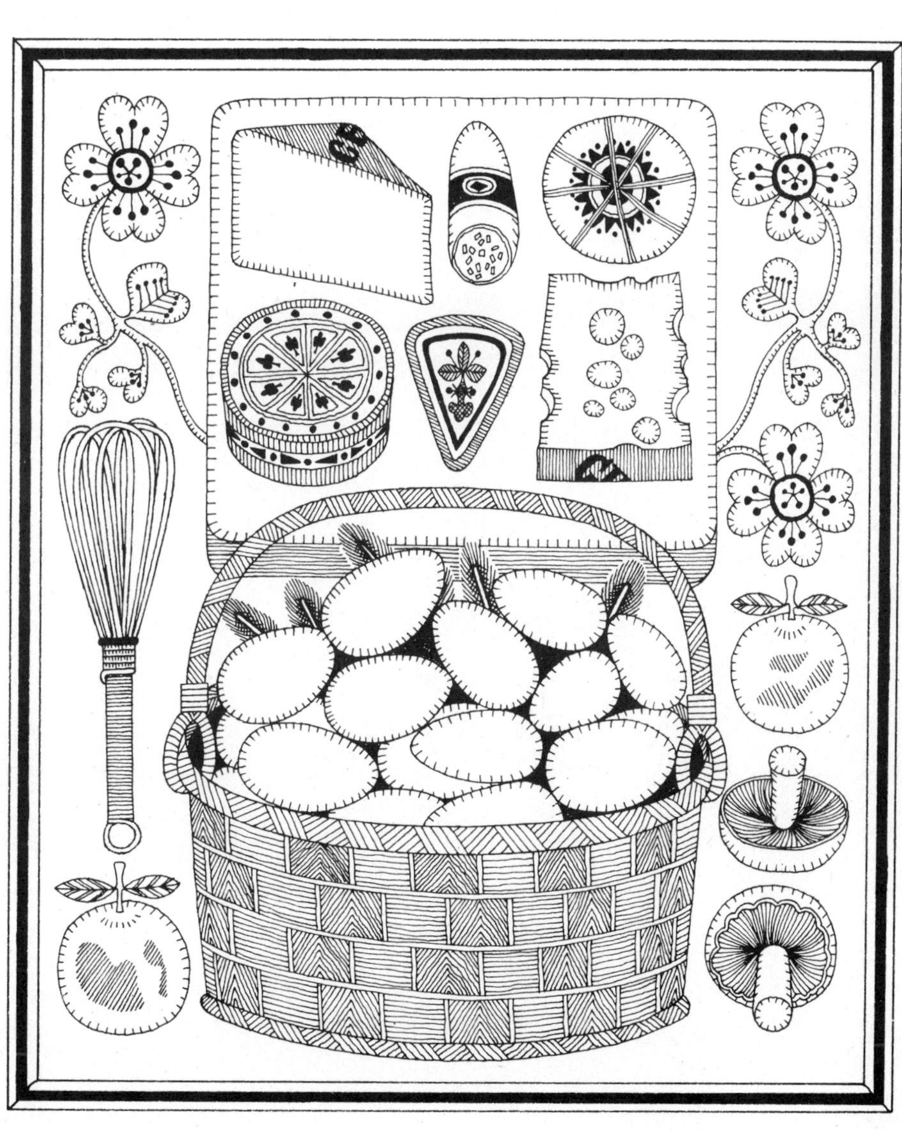

Egg and Cheese Dishes

Eggs and cheese are high in protein value, low in points-count. They're delicious as well as economical. Silhouetters make good use of these excellent foods: just try some of our recipes for size!

CHEESE AND SPINACH CAKES

1–11 ounce packet frozen spinach
¼ ounce butter
4 ounces grated Cheddar cheese
Salt and pepper
Pinch nutmeg
½ egg (beaten)
¼ ounce butter for frying
To coat: beaten egg and browned crumbs

Cook the spinach as directed on the packet. Stir over heat until all the water has evaporated. Stir in butter and cool. Mix in the cheese, seasonings and nutmeg. Beat in the egg. Chill the mixture and then form into 2 round cake shapes about 3 inches in diameter. Coat well with egg and browned crumbs and fry in a little butter about 7 minutes each side until golden brown.

Serves 2

30

CHEESE AND BACON PUDDING

1 egg (separated)
¼ pint slightly warmed milk
2 ounces Cheddar cheese (grated)
1 ounce fresh white bread-crumbs
¼ teaspoon salt
¼ teaspoon dry mustard
2 ounces lean gammon (grilled and chopped)

Beat the egg yolk with the milk and cheese. Mix breadcrumbs with mustard, salt and bacon. Gradually stir in the milk and egg yolk mixture. Leave to stand for 15 minutes. Beat the egg white till it is stiff and then fold into the mixture. Put in a small buttered oven dish and bake in a hot oven (400°F/Gas 6) till golden brown. This should take about 20 minutes. Serve sprinkled with chopped parsley.

Serves 2

27

BACON, MUSHROOM AND ONION LUNCH OMELETTE

2 eggs
3 teaspoons cold water
Salt and pepper
a little butter
1 level tablespoon lean bacon (chopped)
1 level tablespoon mushroom (chopped)
1 level tablespoon onion (chopped)

Beat the eggs with the cold water and add salt and pepper to taste. In a frying pan fry gently in a little butter the bacon, mushroom and onion. Remove from the pan and add to the egg mixture. Heat a little more butter in the pan and cook the omelette mixture as usual.

Serves 2

14

EGG FLORENTINE WITH YOGURT TOPPING

6-ounce packet frozen leaf spinach
2 eggs
Salt and pepper

For topping:
$\frac{1}{2}$ ounce flour
1 5-ounce carton plain yogurt (unsweetened)
1 egg
$\frac{1}{2}$ level tablespoon parmesan cheese (grated)
$\frac{1}{4}$ teaspoon ground nutmeg

Cook spinach according to instructions on packet and drain well. Divide between 2 individual oven dishes. Make a well in the spinach and break an egg into each dish. Season well. Mix together the flour, yogurt and egg for topping and beat until smooth. Divide mixture between dishes pouring carefully over the raw eggs. Sprinkle with parmesan cheese and nutmeg. Bake at 375°F/Gas 5 for 20 minutes until topping is set.

Serves 2

19

COTTAGE CHEESE AND HAM COCOTTES

$\frac{1}{2}$ ounce butter (melted)
4 ounces cottage cheese
1 egg
2 ounces lean boiled ham (chopped)
2 ounces button mushrooms (washed and sliced)
$\frac{1}{2}$ medium onion (finely chopped and softened in a little water and drained)
Salt and pepper
1 tablespoon parsley (freshly chopped)

Brush two individual heat-proof dishes with melted butter. Place on a baking sheet. Beat the cottage cheese and the egg together. Stir in ham, mushrooms, and softened chopped onion, then season to taste. Mix in one tablespoon of chopped parsley. Divide the mixture between the two dishes and cook in a hot oven, 400°F/Gas 6 for 10–15 minutes. Garnish with a little more chopped parsley and serve immediately.

Serves 2

16$\frac{1}{2}$

GARLIC CHEESE APPLE

4 ounces cream cheese (low fat)
1 chive (chopped)
Small piece of garlic (crushed)
$\frac{1}{2}$ teaspoon parsley (chopped)
Seasoning to taste
2 red dessert apples (cored and sliced)
Juice $\frac{1}{2}$ lemon
Lettuce

Mix the cream cheese, chives, garlic, parsley and seasoning together. Toss the apple in the lemon juice to prevent discolouration. Arrange some lettuce leaves on each plate and pipe or spoon a whirl of cream cheese in the centre. Arrange the apple slices round so that they, stand up in the cheese. Serve cold garnished with parsley.

Serves 2

27

EGG AND NUT CURRY

1½ ounces butter
2 ounces onion (chopped)
4 ounces cooking apple (chopped)
2 ounces mushrooms (chopped)
2 ounces mixed roasted nuts (chopped)
¾ level tablespoon curry powder
½ level tablespoon plain flour
¼ pint water
Salt and pepper
2 hard boiled eggs (halved)

Melt butter in a large frying pan, and lightly fry onion, apple and mushrooms for five minutes. Add nuts and lightly fry. Add curry powder and flour, and cook for two minutes, stirring all the time. Gradually add the water and bring to the boil. Season, cover and simmer gently for 30 minutes. Add eggs, cover and simmer for a further 10–15 minutes.

This dish can be served with or without boiled rice, and decorated with parsley or lemon butterflies.

Serves 2

(The illustration shows the dish prepared for 4.)

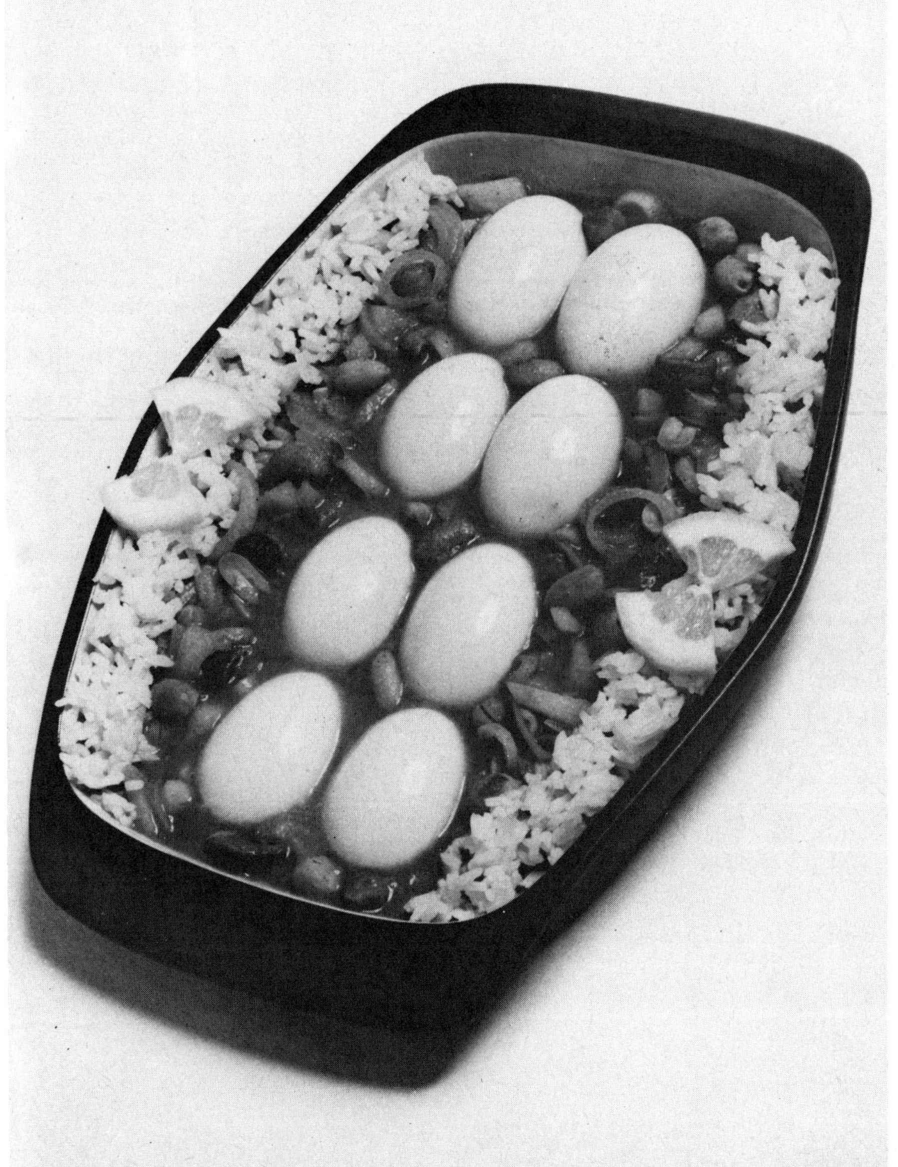

36

HOT CHEESE-STUFFED EGGS

2 hard boiled eggs (shelled)
1 ounce butter (softened)
2 ounces Cheddar cheese (grated)
$\frac{1}{2}$ clove garlic (crushed with a little salt)
Pinch salt and cayenne pepper to taste
$\frac{1}{2}$ tablespoon top of milk

Cheese Sauce:
$\frac{1}{2}$ ounce butter
$\frac{1}{2}$ ounce flour
$\frac{1}{4}$ pint milk
1 ounce Cheddar cheese (grated)
Salt and pepper
$\frac{1}{2}$ ounce Cheddar cheese (extra finely grated)
4 cooked mushroom caps

Cut the hard boiled eggs in half lengthwise, remove yolks and mash with a fork. Add the softened butter, grated cheese, garlic, seasoning and top of the milk and mix well together. Divide the mixture equally between the halved egg whites, piling smoothly, and place in a buttered fireproof dish. Make cheese sauce and coat eggs. Sprinkle with extra grated cheese and brown quickly under a hot grill. Garnish with cooked mushroom caps and serve hot.

Serves 2

39

TORTILLA

2 standard eggs
2 teaspoons cold water
Salt and pepper
1 tablespoon green pepper (chopped)
2 ounces onion (chopped)
$\frac{1}{2}$ tablespoon olive oil

Heat oil in omelette pan, add onion and cook slowly until soft. Add pepper and cook for a few minutes.* Meanwhile, prepare omelette mixture by breaking eggs into a basin, add water and seasonings and beat lightly with a fork, just enough to break up the eggs. Pour this mixture onto the hot onion mixture with the heat high. With a fork or palette knife, stir mixture from sides to the middle of the pan so allowing underside to cook. When this is firm, but the top still runny, set pan under a hot grill for about $\frac{1}{2}$ minute, until just set. Do not fold, but slide out flat onto a warm plate.

* 1 ounce lean chopped ham. Can be added to the onion mixture if liked.

Serves 2

11

SWISS MOUNTAIN OMELETTE

2 standard eggs
2 teaspoons cold water
Salt and pepper
1$\frac{1}{2}$ ounces Cheddar cheese (grated)
1$\frac{1}{2}$ tablespoons double cream
$\frac{1}{2}$ ounce butter

Mix cream and cheese together. Break eggs into a basin, add cold water and season well. Beat together lightly. Place a 6-inch omelette pan over a gentle heat and get thoroughly hot. Add butter and turn up heat. When butter is sizzling hot, pour in egg mixture. Using fork or palette knife, draw setting egg to middle from sides of pan. Repeat until all runny egg is cooked to a soft creamy consistency. Place half the cream and cheese mixture along centre of omelette, fold over one third away from the handle of the pan. Remove from heat and turn out on to a hot fireproof plate, by holding handle of pan with palm uppermost, shaking omelette to edge of pan and tipping over pan to make another fold. Place remaining cream and cheese mixture on top of omelette and put under a very hot grill for a few seconds until top is bubbling and golden. Serve immediately.

Serves 2

24

EGGS EN CASSEROLE

4 ounces cooked smoked fish (e.g, haddock)
2 tablespoons condensed celery soup
1 tablespoon milk
1 tablespoon parsley (chopped)
2 eggs
Salt and pepper
1 ounce Cheddar cheese (grated)

Grease a small ovenproof dish. In a pan heat together all ingredients except eggs and cheese, then place in the dish. Keep warm while the eggs are poached. Place poached eggs on top of mixture, sprinkle with cheese then put under a hot grill until the cheese has melted and the top is golden brown.

Serves 2

19

EGGS PRINCESS

4 ounces mushrooms
2 ounces butter
4 ounces tongue (chopped)
2 teaspoons parsley (chopped)
2 egg yolks
2 tablespoons double cream
2 teaspoons lemon juice
2 eggs
Salt and pepper

Wash and slice mushrooms, fry in 1 ounce butter till soft. Add tongue and most of the parsley. Season to taste. Put in serving dish and keep warm.

In another pan melt remaining butter, add yolks, cream and lemon juice. Stir over low heat until sauce thickens (do not let it boil). Meanwhile fry or poach the eggs. Then pour some sauce over the tongue mixture, put the eggs on top, cover with remaining sauce and sprinkle on the remaining parsley.

Serves 2

50

CAROLINA EGGS

1 rasher lean bacon
2 eggs
Salt and pepper
2 tablespoons sweetcorn (canned or frozen)

Fry bacon till crisp then chop it. Beat the eggs with the seasoning then add bacon and sweetcorn. Heat a little of the bacon fat in a pan, add egg mixture and cook very slowly, as for scrambled eggs. This should be served with a tomato and celery or a green salad.

Serves 2

14

EGGS MORNAY

2 tablespoons onion (chopped)
2 ounces lard
2 tomatoes (peeled, sliced)
2 eggs (hard boiled and sliced)
1 × 6½ ounce can condensed mushroom soup
1 tablespoon milk
2 ounces Cheddar cheese (grated)

Fry onion until soft, but not brown, in lard. Add tomatoes and cook for 2–3 minutes. Transfer mixture to a pie dish then place eggs on top of mixture. Heat soup, milk and 1 ounce of the cheese together in a pan. When hot pour over the eggs. Sprinkle on remaining cheese and place under a hot grill for 2 or 3 minutes until golden brown and bubbling.

Serves 2

48

ORIENTAL EGG SALAD

2 ounces rice
2 ounces raisins
1 small eating apple (cored and chopped)
2 tablespoons celery (chopped)
2 tablespoons cucumber (finely diced, unskinned)
3 tablespoons yogurt salad dressing
1 tablespoon toasted almonds
Paprika pepper and salt
2 hard-boiled eggs (halved lengthwise)

Cook rice in boiling salted water for 12 minutes, strain and cool under cold water. Mix the raisins, apple, celery, cucumber and 1 tablespoon of dressing. Pile on a serving dish. Place eggs, cut side down, on rice mixture and then cover eggs with the rest of the dressing. Sprinkle with almonds and paprika pepper.

Serves 2

31

Meat Dishes

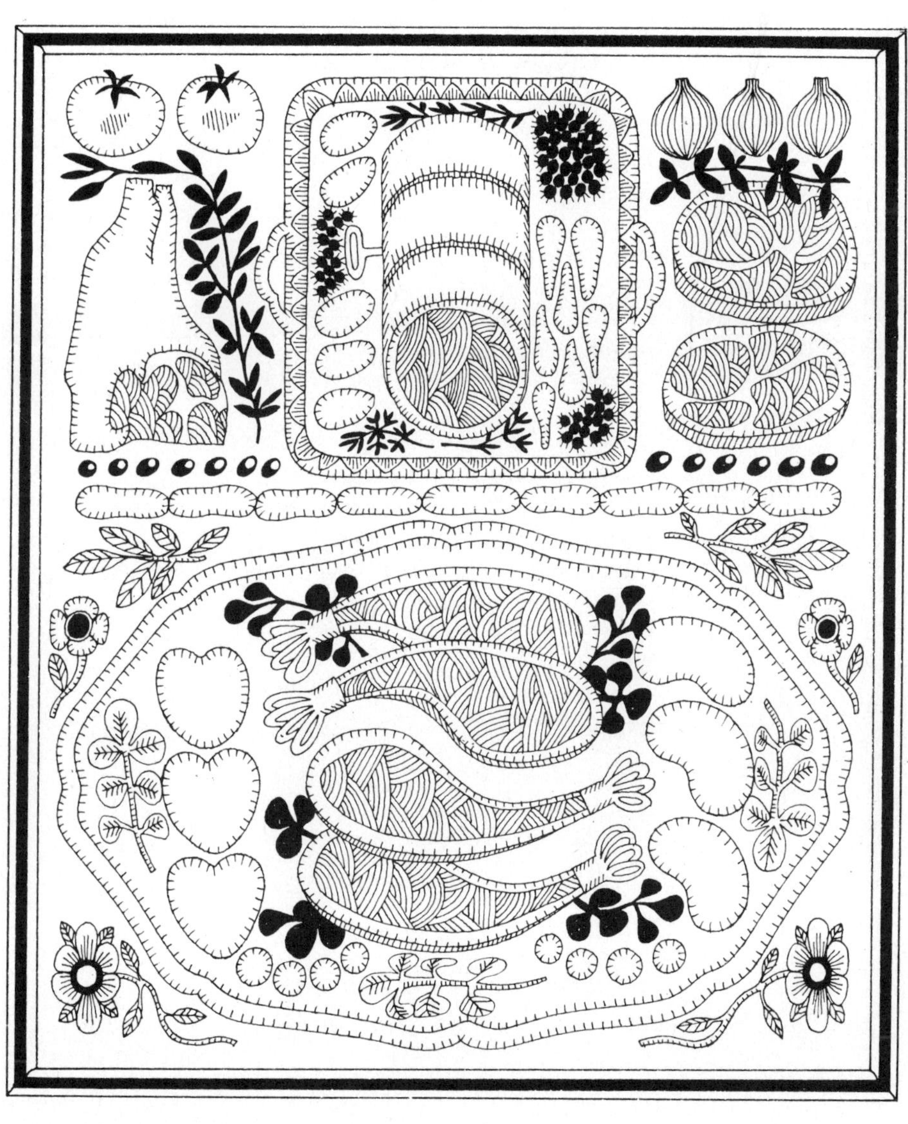

Meat Dishes, including poultry

Most people like meat at least once a day, but there is no reason why this should be expensive. Our meat chapter includes delicious recipes made from the cheaper cuts of meat, as well as some featuring the children's favourite—sausages.

CHICKEN CASSEROLE

6 ounces chicken breast
1 onion (finely chopped)
4 ounces mushrooms (washed and sliced)
2 tomatoes (sliced)
1 pint stock
Pinch cayenne pepper
Pinch paprika pepper
Salt to taste

If the chicken is already cooked, this dish will only take half the stated cooking time. Place the chicken in a casserole dish with the onions, mushrooms and tomatoes. Season to taste and add the cayenne and paprika pepper. Cook slowly in oven 300°F/Gas 2 for three hours.

Serves 2

16½

STUFFED HEARTS

2 lambs' hearts

Stuffing:
2 ounces streaky bacon
2 ounces fresh breadcrumbs
½ tablespoon parsley (chopped)
1 ounce sultanas
2 teaspoons grated lemon rind
Seasoning
½ ounce butter
½ small egg (beaten)
Seasoned flour
1 small tin tomato juice

Prepare and trim the hearts. Mince or chop the bacon and add all the remaining ingredients and mix well. keeping back the tomato juice. Stuff each heart and secure the top with a cocktail stick. Toss in seasoned flour and brown all over in fat. Place in a casserole dish, pour over the tomato juice and bake for 1½ hours at 350°F/Gas 4.
Slice hearts before serving.

Serves 2

48

SAUSAGE AND ONION WEDGES

1 tomato
6 ounces beef sausage meat
1 egg
¼ pint milk
1 tablespoon parsley (chopped)
1 heaped tablespoon onion (finely chopped)
Salt and pepper

Skin and slice the tomato. Line a small flan case or shallow cake tin with sausage meat about ½-inch thick. Beat egg, stir in milk, parsley, onion and seasoning. Pour into sausage case and top with slices of tomato. Bake at 400°F/Gas 6 until the custard is set and sausage meat cooked, about ½ hour. Serve hot or cold cut into wedges.

Serves 2

44

SPRING LAMB ROAST

1 breast lamb, boned and trimmed (approx. 1 pound)

Stuffing:
½ ounce butter or margarine
1 small onion (finely chopped)
½ small lemon
1 tablespoon fresh mint (chopped)
3 ounces fresh breadcrumbs
½ beaten egg
Salt and pepper

Sauce:
⅛ pint vinegar
1 tablespoon mint (chopped)
1 teaspoon caster sugar
½ tablespoon honey
½ teaspoon soy sauce
½ level tablespoon cornflour
⅛ pint water

Melt the butter in a pan, add onion and cook gently for five minutes. Grate rind from lemon then discard pith and cut flesh into ¼-inch cubes. Add to remaining stuffing ingredients with onion and mix well. Spread stuffing over meat. Roll up and secure with string. Sprinkle with salt and pepper. Place in a roasting pan and cook at 400°F/Gas 6 for about ¾ hour, or until meat is cooked.

Place all ingredients, except cornflour and water, in a pan and bring to the boil. Blend cornflour with water. Stir into sauce, bring to the boil, stirring all the time, and cook for 1 minute. Just before serving, stir meat juices from tin into sauce. Serve sauce separately.

Serves 4

116

BEEF CASSEROLE AND DUMPLINGS

½ pound stewing steak
3 small carrots (sliced)
2 small tomatoes (sliced)
Parsley
Thyme and bayleaf
Seasoning
1 sliced onion (large)
Flour (to thicken)
½ pint water
⅛ pint dry cider
Little fat

Dumplings:
1 ounce self-raising flour
1 ounce fresh breadcrumbs
1 ounce suet
1 dessertspoon mixed herbs
Salt and pepper to taste

Casserole: Cut the stewing steak into 1-inch cubes. Sauté in the fat until browned on all sides. Remove and add the onion and carrots. Fry for 2–3 minutes. Stir in the flour and then add the water and the cider. Bring to the boil and add the herbs, seasoning and the meat. Turn into a casserole dish and bake for 1¼ hours at 350°F/Gas 4.

Dumplings:
Mix all the dry ingredients together and bind with a little water to form a soft dough. Divide into two equal portions and form into two rounds approximately 2–3 inches wide. Place on top of the casserole and cook for 25 minutes.

Serves 2

49

ITALIAN STUFFED MEAT ROLLS

2 slices silverside or 2 'flash fry' steaks (approx 1 pound)
2 rashers back bacon

Stuffing
1 medium onion (finely chopped)
1 ounce butter
$\frac{1}{2}$ tablespoon oil
1 ounce Cheddar cheese (grated)
$\frac{1}{2}$ teaspoon marjoram
$\frac{1}{2}$ ounce sultanas
$\frac{1}{2}$ ounce blanched almonds (chopped)
Salt and pepper

For braising:
$\frac{1}{2}$ tablespoon oil
1 tablespoon tomato purée
$\frac{1}{2}$ pint stock or water
Salt and pepper

Trim off any excess fat from meat. Lay on a board and flatten with a rolling pin until very thin. Fry bacon gently for one minute on each side then place a rasher on each slice of meat.

Stuffing: Cook onions gently in butter and oil without browning for 3–4 minutes. Remove half the onions and keep on one side. Add rest of stuffing ingredients to remaining onion and mix well. Divide equally between meat slices and press down. Roll up tightly and secure ends with cocktail sticks.

80

To Braise: Heat oil in frying pan. Brown meat rolls evenly on all sides. Add remaining onion and tomato purée mixed with stock or water, season and bring to the boil. Place meat and sauce in a casserole. Bake in a low oven, 300°F/Gas 2 for 45 minutes until meat is tender.

Serves 4

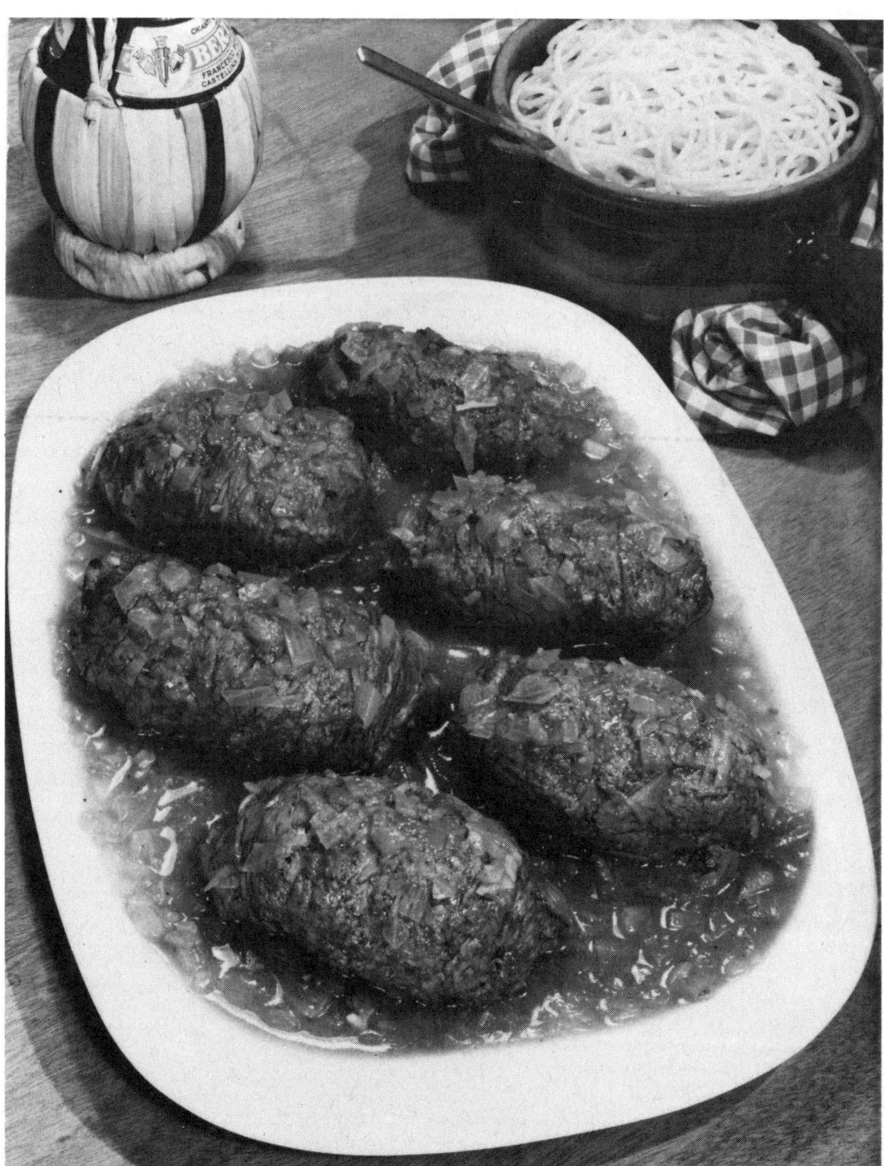

MINCE COBBLER

1 onion
1 ounce lard
2 ounces ox kidney
6 ounces minced beef
1 ounce flour
1 ounce mushrooms
1 carrot (grated)
Seasoning
1 bouillon cube (crumbled and dissolved in $\frac{1}{2}$ pint hot water)

Topping:
4 ounces plain flour
1 teaspoon baking powder
1 ounce butter
Milk to mix

Dice the onion and sauté in hot fat. Coarsely chop the kidney, combine it with the mince and cook gently. Stir in the flour; add the sliced mushroom, grated carrot, seasoning and bouillon stock. Make up the topping, using the rubbing-in method, and add enough milk to form a soft but not sticky dough. Knead lightly and roll out to $\frac{1}{2}$-inch thick, cut into shapes and place on top of mince. Brush with milk. Cover with a sheet of greaseproof paper and cook at 375°F/Gas 5 for approximately 25 minutes, or until golden brown.

Serves 2

64

BEEF ELDORADO

1 tablespoon oil
1 small onion (thickly sliced)
2 carrots (cut in $\frac{1}{2}$-inch lengths)
$\frac{1}{2}$ pound beef chuck steak
Seasoned flour
$\frac{1}{3}$ pint light ale
1 dessertspoon black treacle
1 ounce sultanas
Seasoning

Heat the oil and fry the onion and carrots for two minutes. Add the beef, cubed and tossed in seasoned flour. Fry until the meat is coloured. Pour the light ale into the pan and bring to the boil. Add the treacle and sultanas. Cover and cook at 325°F/Gas 3, for about 1$\frac{1}{2}$–2 hours. Serve with natural yogurt, sprinkled with chopped parsley, noodles and a green vegetable (additional points, *see* pp. 102–106).

Serves 2

42

SAVOURY PLAIT

1 tablespoon oil
$\frac{1}{2}$ onion (chopped)
4 ounces minced beef
Tabasco sauce
$\frac{1}{2}$ tablespoon tube tomato paste
Pinch mixed herbs
2 ounces mixed vegetables (cooked and diced, with seasoning)
1 × 7$\frac{1}{2}$-ounce packet frozen puff pastry
Beaten egg to glaze

Heat the oil and gently fry the onion and the beef. Add a shake of Tabasco sauce with the tomato paste, herbs, vegetables and seasoning. Mix well and set aside to cool slightly. Roll out the thawed pastry to a rectangle about 10 inches × 6 inches. Place filling lengthways down the centre. Make slanting cuts $\frac{1}{2}$-inch apart down the length of the pastry on either side of filling. Bring strips up to the centre alternately to give a plaited effect. Brush with beaten egg and bake at 425°F/Gas 7, for about 25 minutes. Serve hot or cold.

Serves 2

55$\frac{1}{2}$

COSMOPOLITAN STEAK

2 ounces onion (finely sliced)
Dripping for frying
2 × 6–8 ounce pieces
Argentine beef (topside, top rump or chuck steak)
1 ounce flour
Salt and pepper
½ pint beef stock
1 dessertspoon vinegar
½ teaspoon made mustard
½ teaspoon paprika
½ teaspoon thyme

Garnish:
Onion rings (raw or canned)
Parsley sprigs

Fry sliced onion in heated dripping until brown. Place in a casserole dish. Dip pieces of beef in seasoned flour and fry them in a little more dripping until a light brown on both sides. Add to the onions. Stir most of the remaining flour into the pan and fry until nut brown. Add the stock, vinegar, mustard, paprika and thyme and bring to the boil, stirring. Season and pour over the steak. Cover the casserole with a lid and place in the oven at 300°F–325°F/Gas 2–3, adjusting temperature if necessary so that casserole simmers slowly. Cook for 1½ hours approximately, or until the meat is tender. To serve, place the pieces of steak on a hot dish and pour the sauce over them. Serve extra sauce separately. Garnish with onion rings and sprigs of parsley.

Serves 2

54½

BEEF WITH NOODLES

3 ounces dry noodles
2 tablespoons oil
½ pound minced beef
4 tablespoons onion (chopped)
½ clove garlic
3 medium tomatoes
½ pint stock or water
2 sticks celery (if available)
1 green pepper (finely chopped)
Salt and pepper

Sauce:
1 teaspoon cornflour
2 teaspoons soy sauce
3 tablespoons water

Cook the noodles in boiling salted water, when tender, drain and set aside to keep hot. Using a heavy frying pan, heat the cooking oil, but do not let it discolour. Add the minced beef, onion, crushed garlic and chopped tomatoes. Simmer for five minutes, stirring it constantly to prevent sticking. Pour in the stock and add the diced celery and the finely chopped green pepper. Cover the pan and let this mixture simmer for five minutes more. Taste and add the seasoning.

Meanwhile, mix the sauce ingredients and add to the pan. Reduce the heat and simmer five minutes more to allow the sauce to richen and thicken. Arrange the hot noodles on a dish and pour the meat and sauce over. Serve hot.

Serves 2

53

GOLDEN HOT POT

1 small onion
2 ounces mushrooms
6 ounces middle neck of lamb
Salt
Pepper
$\frac{1}{4}$ pint stock

Place alternate layers of onion, mushrooms and middle neck of lamb in a fireproof dish, seasoning well between layers. Pour in stock, cover with kitchen foil and cook in moderately slow oven (325°F/Gas 3) for about $1\frac{1}{2}$ hours or till tender.

Serves 2

14

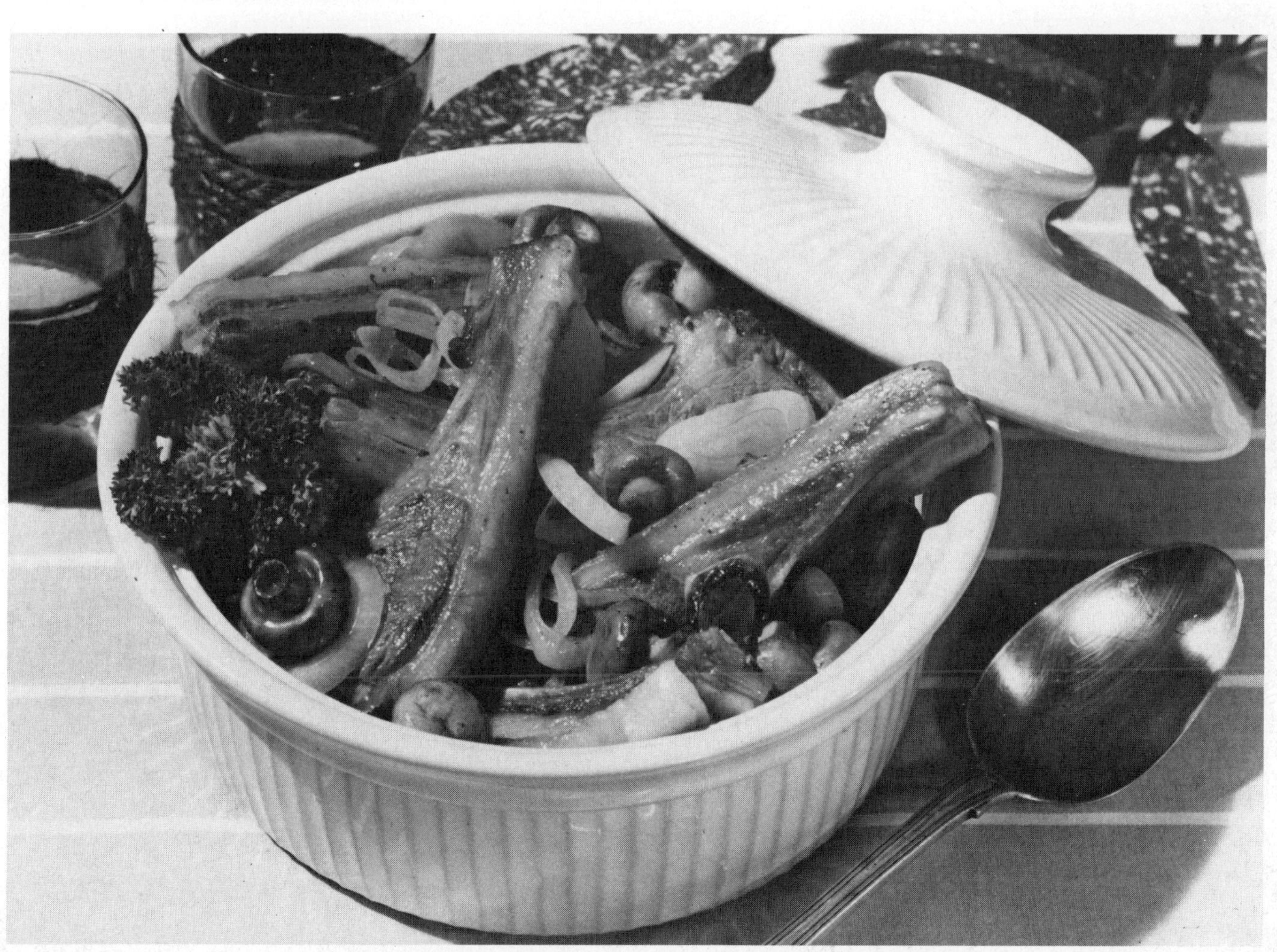

PIQUANT HORSERADISH CASSEROLE

Béchamel Sauce:
½ pint milk
small onion stuck with 4 cloves
Small carrot
Parsley stalks
1 bayleaf
2–3 peppercorns
Pinch ground mace
¾ ounce butter
1 level tablespoon flour
Seasoning
1 tablespoon oil

1 small onion (sliced)
¾ pound beef (Forerib or Topside)
½ green pepper (cut in strips)
2 ounces mushrooms (quartered)
2 teaspoons horseradish relish

To make the Béchamel Sauce, pour the milk into a pan and bring gently to the boil with the onion, carrot, parsley, bayleaf, peppercorns and mace. Remove from heat and allow flavours to infuse for approximately 30 minutes. Melt the butter in a pan, stir in the flour and cook until golden and foaming. Remove from heat and gradually stir in the strained milk. Bring to the boil stirring well. Season to taste. Heat the oil and gently fry the sliced onion. Meanwhile cut the beef into thin strips, ½ inch × 1½ inches. Add to the onion and fry gently. Stir in the prepared green pepper and mushrooms and leave on a gentle heat. Add Béchamel Sauce and horseradish relish. Cover and cook at 325°F/Gas 3 for 1 hour. Serve on rice sprinkled with chopped parsley.

Serves 4

59

SPICY BEEF CASSEROLE

¾ pound chuck steak or brisket of beef
1 ounce butter
1 large onion (sliced)
½ clove garlic (crushed or finely chopped)
½ pint stock or water
1 glass dry red wine
½ pound carrots (sliced)
½ level dessertspoon tomato purée
Bouquet garni
Pinch ground mace
¼ level teaspoon caraway seeds
Salt and pepper
4 ounces large mushrooms (thickly sliced)
½ level tablespoon plain flour

Cut meat into cubes, removing any excess fat. Melt butter in a large pan. Brown the meat all over and lightly fry the onion and garlic. Add the stock, wine, carrots, tomato purée, bouquet garni, mace, caraway seeds and seasoning. Cover and simmer for about 2 hours. Add the mushrooms and continue cooking for a further 30 minutes. Using a draining spoon, transfer the meat and vegetables to a casserole or serving dish and keep hot. Remove the bouquet garni. Blend flour with a little water and stir into the liquid in the pan. Bring to the boil, stirring all the time, and cook for a minute. Season again if necessary, and pour over the meat.

Serves 4

55

ISLAND BEEF

- $\frac{1}{2}$ pound tender lean beef (cut into 1-inch cubes)
- 1 tablespoon soy sauce
- 1 tablespoon dry white wine
- 1 tablespoon corn oil
- Pepper
- 1 clove garlic
- Small tin water chestnuts (drained)
- 1 red or green pepper (cut into strips)

Marinate beef chunks for at least half an hour in soy sauce, white wine and corn oil, seasoned with pepper and mashed garlic. Thread on skewers with water chestnuts and green or red pepper slices and cook over charcoal or under grill until tender, turning frequently and basting with the marinade.

Serves 2

36

VEAL CUTLETS PAPILLOTE

- $\frac{1}{4}$ pound onions
- 1 small garlic clove
- 2 large tomatoes
- Pinch dried thyme
- Salt and pepper
- 2 ounces butter
- 2 veal cutlets or escalopes

Peel onion and chop finely, crush garlic clove, skin and chop the tomatoes and place these ingredients in a small heavy pan. Add thyme, salt and pepper to taste and if the tomatoes are under-ripe or dry, add about a tablespoon of stock. Cover, cook gently for about five minutes, then uncover and cook to a thick sauce, stirring occasionally to prevent sticking.

Sauté the veal in the butter until brown, turning once. Cut oblongs of greaseproof paper large enough to envelop each escalope or cutlet. Butter greaseproof paper lightly. Divide half the tomato mixture between two pieces of buttered greaseproof paper. Season veal slices with salt and pepper, put on top of tomato mixture, spread each with half the remaining tomato mixture.

Draw up sides of greaseproof paper and form into an envelope, fold ends to seal. Place on baking sheet in centre of hot oven, 400°F/Gas 6, and cook for about 10 minutes. Lift carefully to avoid paper splitting and losing all the juice.

Serves 2

32$\frac{1}{2}$

BOSTON CASSEROLE

- 1 pound belly pork
- 3 ounces haricot beans (soaked overnight)
- 1 stalk celery (sliced)
- 1 large carrot (sliced)
- $\frac{1}{4}$ teaspoon mustard (dry)
- $\frac{1}{2}$ tablespoon sugar
- $\frac{1}{2}$ tablespoon golden syrup
- Stock cube dissolved in $\frac{1}{3}$ pint hot water

Soak haricot beans overnight. Place pork in casserole, surround with beans and other vegetables. Mix the dry mustard, sugar and syrup with the stock and seasoning. Pour into casserole. Cover with lid and bake at 350°F/Gas 4 for approximately 2$\frac{1}{2}$ hours. Half an hour before casserole is ready to be served, remove lid to crisp the outside of the pork. Garnish with chopped parsley and lemon butterflies.

Serves 4

10

KEBABS

Uncooked meat (any)
Button or quartered mushrooms
Green pepper
2 tomatoes (quartered)
Salt
Pepper
Bayleaves

Thread small cubes of uncooked meat, a few mushrooms, pieces of green pepper, bayleaves and quartered tomatoes onto a skewer. Season and brush with oil. Place under medium grill until cooked, turning frequently.

10 (for 3 skewers)

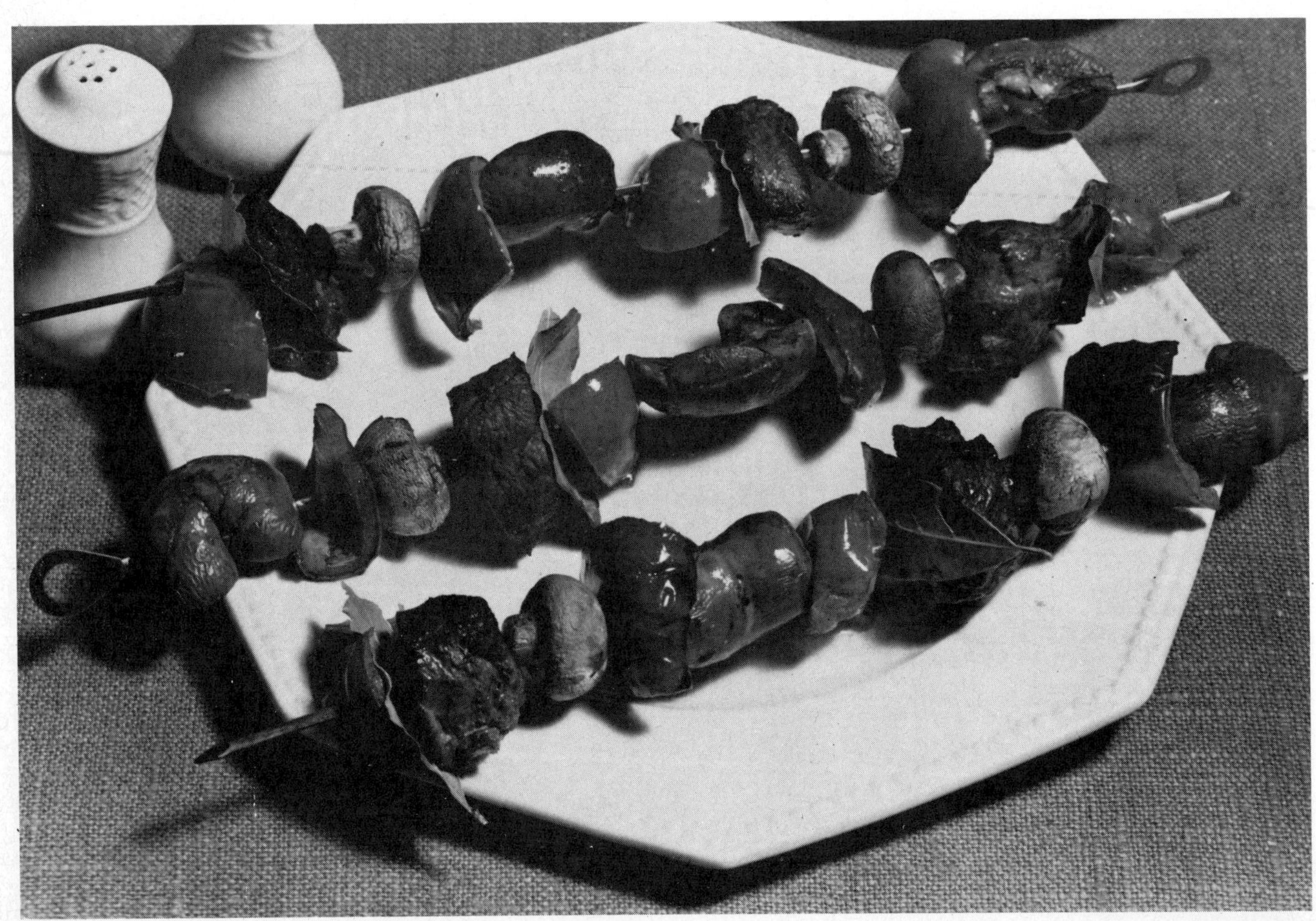

LIVER CASSEROLE

$\frac{1}{2}$ pound pig's liver
4 ounces onions
1 ounce carrots (grated)
4 ounces leeks
Salt and pepper
$\frac{1}{4}$ teaspoon sage
$\frac{1}{2}$ pint stock

Chop the liver and place in a lightly greased casserole in the oven, 350°F/Gas 4 for 15 minutes, stirring occasionally. Meanwhile, peel the onion and chop it roughly. Wash, scrape and grate the carrot; remove the outer leaves and roots of leeks, halve lengthwise and cut into 4-inch strips, wash thoroughly. Heat the stock. Remove the liver from the oven. Add the vegetables, seasonings, sage and boiling stock and return to the oven. Simmer until the liver is cooked and most of the stock has been absorbed. Remove from oven and place the meat on a warm dish. Should any stock remain, strain from the vegetables and put these through a sieve. Cover the meat with the vegetable purée and sprinkle with parsley just before serving.

Serves 2

16

BLAND BOILED BACON

1 small (1$\frac{1}{4}$-pound approx.) bacon joint
1 tablespoon Golden Syrup
6 peppercorns
1 bayleaf
$\frac{3}{4}$ pint water

Put bacon joint into a small saucepan. Add syrup, peppercorns, bayleaf and water. Bring to the boil then cover with a lid and reduce heat so that bacon simmers gently for about 1 hour. This can be served hot or cold.

Serves 4

95$\frac{1}{2}$

STUFFED CABBAGE LEAVES

2 large cabbage leaves
1 ounce butter
1 onion (chopped)
3 ounces calves liver (chopped)
$\frac{1}{2}$ tablespoon tomato purée
Salt and pepper
Small pinch nutmeg

Place cabbage leaves in a large saucepan and cover with cold water. Bring water just to the boil and remove pan from the heat. Leave standing for five minutes and then drain and dry. Fry the onions in the butter until it is soft but not brown. Add the chopped liver and fry for five minutes. Stir in the tomato purée, water, nutmeg and seasonings. Cool slightly. Divide the filling between the cabbage leaves, fold up tightly into parcels and place in a fireproof dish. Bake in a moderate oven, 350°F/Gas 4, for about an hour.

Serves 2

15$\frac{1}{2}$

KIDNEYS IN PIQUANT SAUCE

4 lambs' kidneys (12 ounces)
$\frac{1}{4}$ pint beef stock
2 ounces mushrooms (sliced)
$\frac{1}{2}$ tablespoon tomato purée
1 teaspoon prepared English mustard
$\frac{1}{2}$ carton natural yogurt (unsweetened)
Salt and pepper to taste

Pour boiling water onto the kidneys and allow to soak for half an hour. Skin, cut in half and remove the core. Place in a pan with the stock, mushrooms, and tomato purée. Cook, covered for 20 minutes or until tender. Stir in mustard and yogurt. Season to taste. Sprinkle with parsley before serving.

Serves 2

18$\frac{1}{2}$

GRILLED GAMMON AND ORANGE

2 medium gammon steaks
1 large orange
$\frac{1}{2}$ ounce butter
$\frac{1}{2}$ ounce demerara sugar
Pepper

Snip the rind of the gammon steaks at intervals to prevent them curling up. Remove peel and all the pith from the orange and cut it into four slices. Dot the steaks with butter and put under a very hot grill for five minutes. Remove from the grill, turn, and sprinkle with sugar. Put under the grill again for a further five minutes. Before returning to the grill to cook the second side, add the orange slices to the grill. Before serving spoon the juices over the gammon steaks and serve with the orange slices.

Serves 2

23$\frac{1}{2}$

LIVER HOT POT

4 ounces liver
4 rashers bacon (lean)
$\frac{1}{4}$ pound mushrooms
2 tomatoes
Medium onion (sliced)

Place the bacon on a sheet of foil, one for each person. Place liver on top of bacon and cover with sliced mushrooms, sliced onion and sliced tomato. Carefully pinch the edges of the foil into paper bag shape so that the juices cannot escape, and put the parcels on the highest shelf in the oven at 375°F/Gas 5 for $\frac{1}{2}$ hour. Pour the juices into a container when the dish is cooked and use in the evening with a teaspoon of beef extract as a hunger bar.

Serves 2

29

MEAT LOAF

1½ ounces soft margarine
6 ounces onions (peeled and diced)
3 ounces mushrooms (peeled and diced)
1 ounce plain flour
6 fluid ounces milk
2 large eggs
1 teaspoon Worcestershire sauce
1 teaspoon salt
¾ teaspoon mixed herbs
3 tablespoons tomato purée
1 tablespoon parmesan cheese
1 tablespoon parsley (chopped)
1 pound minced beef
6 ounces lean minced pork
3 ounces white breadcrumbs

Melt the margarine in a medium saucepan. Fry diced onion till soft, but not brown, then add mushrooms and cook for a further minute. Add flour and milk and, whisking continuously over a moderate heat, bring to the boil and continue cooking for 2–3 minutes. Pour the cooked mixture into a mixing bowl and allow to cool slightly. Add all remaining ingredients and stir together till well mixed. Place in a greased 2-pound loaf tin and bake in a moderate oven 350°F/Gas 4 for 1–1¼ hours. Cool slightly then turn out onto a wire tray. When cold, wrap the loaf in greaseproof paper and chill in the refrigerator. Decorate with slices of hard-boiled egg and cucumber before serving with a green salad.

Serves 8

117

CREAMY CORNED BEEF RISSOLES

1 small can evaporated milk
2 ounces flour
2 ounces butter
1 (12-ounce) can corned beef
1 small onion (grated)
Salt and pepper
2–3 drops Worcestershire sauce
1 egg (beaten)
1 tablespoon flour
breadcrumbs for coating
Little oil for frying

Make up the evaporated milk to ½ pint with water. Whisk in flour and place in a saucepan with the butter. Stir constantly over a moderate heat until the sauce boils and thickens. Mash corned beef with a fork and add to the sauce with the onion. Season to taste with salt and pepper and add Worcestershire sauce. Spread mixture over a plate and leave until cold and firm. Divide into twelve and mould into rissole shape. Coat with flour, dip in beaten egg and roll in breadcrumbs. Fry in deep hot fat until golden brown. Drain well and serve hot.

Serves 4

94

BEEF ROLLS

2 thin slices topside beef (about 4 — 6 inches)
2 rashers streaky bacon (chopped)
½ onion (chopped)
¾ teaspoon mustard powder
¾ teaspoon salt
Pinch pepper
Flour
Cooking fat or oil
½ pint beef stock

Pound the beef slices. Mix together the bacon, onion, mustard powder. Season beef slices and spread with the bacon mixture. Roll up tightly and secure with cocktail sticks. Dredge with a little flour, then brown in hot oil or fat. Pour beef stock over rolls in pan, cover and simmer for 30 minutes. Remove from pan and keep hot. Add ½ tablespoon flour moistened with a little water and cook until thickened, stirring all the time. Pour gravy over beef rolls and serve.

Serves 2

32

DEVILLED KIDNEYS

4 lambs' kidneys
2 tablespoons butter
Salt and pepper
½ teaspoon curry powder
2 rashers steaky bacon (rolled)

Skin kidneys, then remove core and wash and dry well. Slice almost through the middle. Open out flat and secure with a skewer. Brush one side with melted butter and sprinkle with salt, pepper and half the curry powder. Cook under grill slowly on one side (approximately 5 minutes). Turn kidneys and brush again with butter, season again. Grill slowly till tender. Grill the bacon rolls during the last few minutes of cooking.

Serves 2

39½

STEAK SUISSE

1 tablespoon oil
1 onion (peeled and sliced)
½ lb chuck steak
Bay leaf
Salt and pepper
4 tomatoes (skinned and chopped)
1 tablespoon tomato purée

Heat the oil in a pan and sauté the onions until tender but not brown. Cut steak into pieces and brown it in the oil. Add the chopped tomatoes and tomato purée and stir well. Add bay leaf and seasoning. Place in a casserole, cover and cook for 2 hours or until meat is tender at 350°F/Gas 4.

Serves 2

33½

O'FLANAGAN'S SAUSAGE SUPPER

½ pound beef sausages
1 large onion (peeled and cut into rings)
1 ounce lard
Seasoning
2 small red-skinned apples (cored and cut into rings)
Parsley for garnish

Grill the sausages until just cooked, but not too brown. Sauté the onions in the lard until transparent, add the apple rings and toss together. Season to taste. Place the sausages, apple rings and onion in a shallow ovenproof dish and bake in a moderately hot oven, 400°F/ Gas 6 for 20 minutes.

Serves 2

47

SPICY SAUSAGE POT

1 packet oxtail soup
1 pint water
8 ounces sausages (cooked)
2 ounces peas (cooked or frozen)
3 sticks celery (finely chopped)
1 dessert apple (chopped)
Salt and pepper
¼ teaspoon chilli powder

Make up the oxtail soup with the pint of water. Add the sausages, thickly sliced, the peas, celery, chopped apple, and chili powder. Season to taste. Stir well and simmer for five minutes.

Serves 2

41

SYDNEY STYLE SAUSAGES

½ pound pork sausages
½ ounce butter
2 ounces Cheddar cheese (grated)
½ egg
½ teaspoon Continental mustard

Place the sausages in a saucepan and cover with cold water. Slowly bring to the boil. Drain and place under the grill. Grill for ten minutes. Meanwhile, prepare the topping. Melt the butter and remove from the heat. Add grated cheese, egg and mustard. Mix well together. When sausages are cooked, split and spoon topping over them. Place under the grill until golden brown. Serve with grilled tomatoes.

Serves 2

50½

SPICED FRANKFURTERS AND FRUIT

6 ounces frankfurters
2 tablespoons fruit chutney
2 tablespoons spiced wine vinegar
Small pinch powdered ginger
Small pinch grated nutmeg
1 teaspoon lemon rind (finely grated)
Seasoning
1 pear (peeled, cored and sliced)
Juice one lemon
Seasoning
2 ounces glacé apricots (cut in halves)

To serve: plain boiled rice (points extra)

Place the frankfurters in a saucepan with the chutney, vinegar, wine, spices and lemon rind. Heat together for five minutes. Season to taste. Toss the pear slices in lemon juice and add to the saucepan with the glacé apricots. Simmer for a further 5–8 minutes. Serve on a bed of rice.

Serves 2

27½

SAUSAGE HOT POT

½ pound beef sausage meat
1 pound potatoes (peeled and thinly sliced)
2 onions (thinly sliced)
8-ounce can tomatoes
½ pint stock (made with stock cube)
Salt and pepper

Roll the sausage meat into small balls, and fry until they are golden brown all over. Remove from the pan and drain on absorbent paper. Place all the ingredients in layers in a casserole, finishing with a layer of potatoes. Pour over the stock and add salt and pepper. Cover and cook for 1½ hours at 375°F/Gas 5. Half an hour before the end of the cooking time, remove the lid and allow the potatoes to brown.

Serves 2

69

CHICKEN AND PRAWN CAPRI

2 chicken joints (uncooked)
3 ounce prawns
1 green or red pepper (chopped)
1 onion (chopped)
1 ounce butter
Seasoning to taste
Bouquet garni
1 pint stock
A little cornflour to thicken

Chop the chicken into bite-sized pieces. Sauté gently in the butter for a few minutes, add chopped peppers and stock. Simmer until tender (about 1 hour) with bouquet garni. When tender, remove bouquet garni and add prawns. Cook for a further 15 minutes. If liked, thicken gravy with cornflour mixed to a thin paste with a little water. Serve with salad or boiled rice (points extra).

Serves 2

36

CHICKEN WITH LEMON BUTTER

4 chicken joints
Salt
Pepper
3 ounces butter
1 teaspoon oil
Juice 1 lemon
2 bayleaves
Chopped parsley
Lemon slices

Wipe the chicken and season well. Heat 2 ounces butter with the oil in frying pan and fry the joints till golden brown all over and cooked through (about 15–20 minutes). Place the chicken on a hot serving dish and keep hot. Add remaining butter to the pan. When hot add the lemon juice and the bayleaves and boil for a short while. Pour over the chicken, sprinkle with parsley and garnish with lemon slices.

Serves 4

14

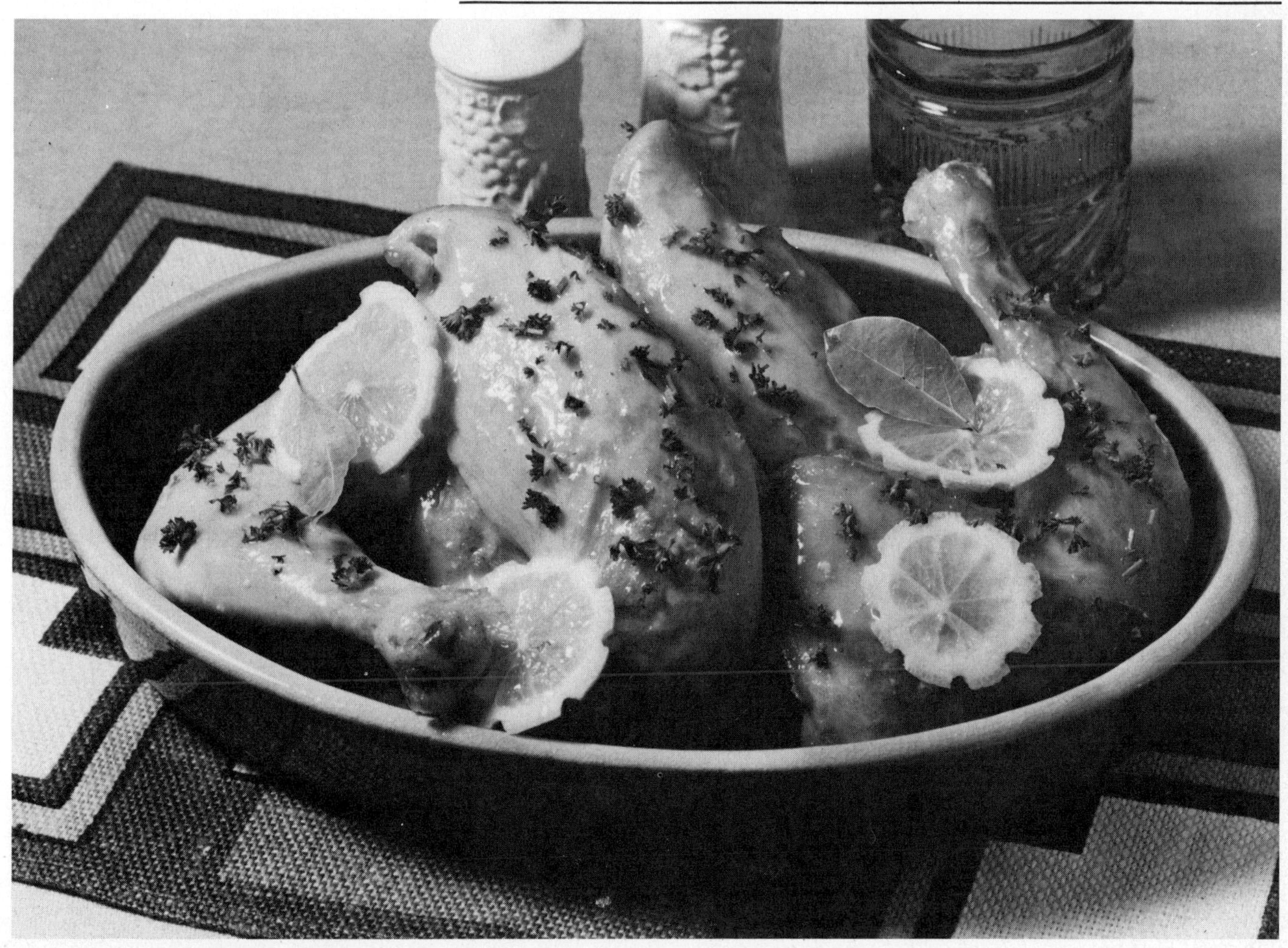

HAWAIIAN CHICKEN

1 tablespoon corn oil
2 ounces blanched sliced almonds
1 large onion (sliced)
1 packet mushroom soup
¼ pint milk
¾ pint water
1 pound cooked chicken (cut into pieces)
8-ounce tin of pineapple titbits (drained)

Heat the oil in a pan and lightly brown the almonds. Remove almonds, and sauté the onion in the remaining oil until tender. Add 1 packet mushroom soup, milk and water. Bring to the boil, stirring all the time. Add the chicken, pineapple and the almonds. Mix well and simmer gently for 15 minutes. This can be served alone or with plain boiled rice (points extra).

Serves 4

74

CHICKEN AND TOMATO BAKE

2 ounces mushrooms
1 ounce butter or margarine
1 medium onion (finely chopped)
2 chicken joints
1 ounce seasoned flour
1 medium tomato (sliced)
Small can condensed kidney soup
½ can water
Seasoning

Gently fry mushrooms in melted butter until tender, remove from pan. Fry onion until tender and golden brown. Add the chicken joints, coated with seasoned flour, and fry until brown on all sides. Place onion, chicken, mushrooms and tomatoes in a greased shallow ovenproof dish. Blend the soup with the water and seasoning and pour over chicken. Cover well and bake in a moderate oven, 350°F/Gas 4 for 1 hour.

Serves 2

32

Fish Dishes

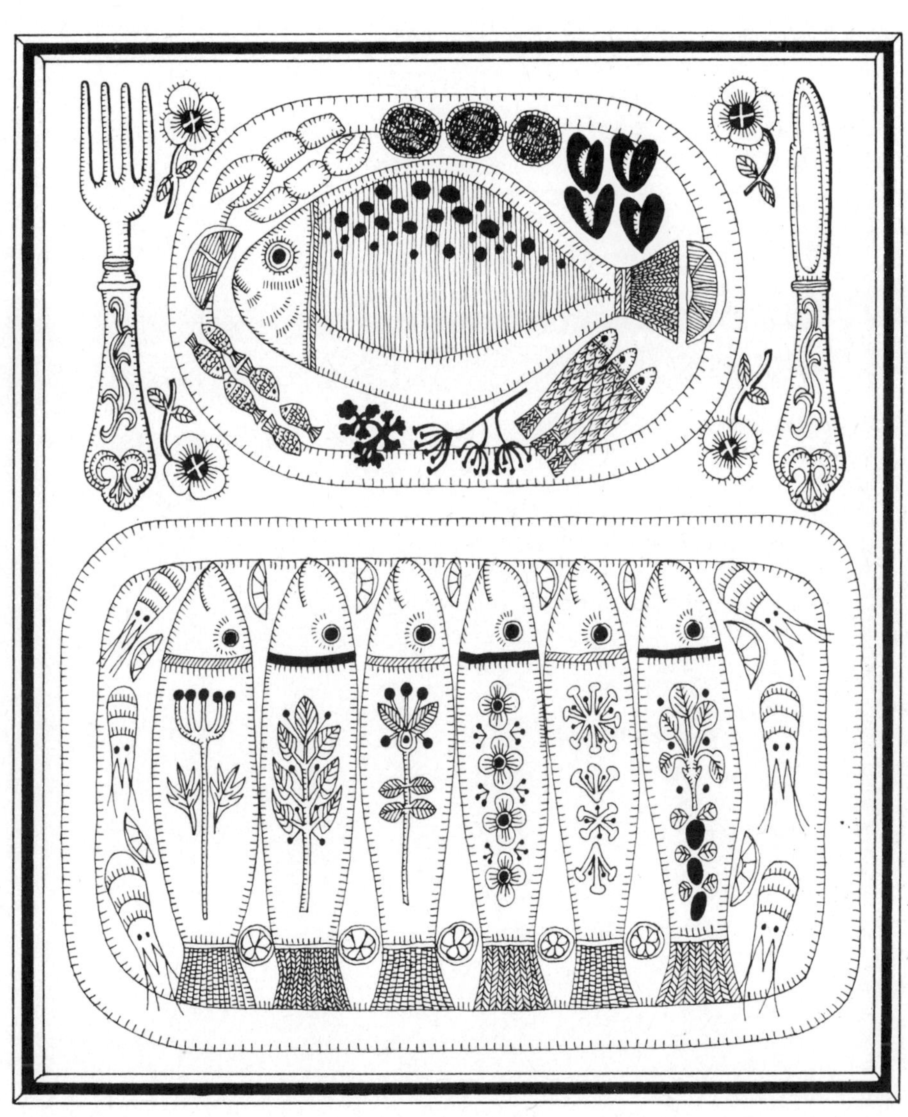

Fish Dishes

'Fish and chips' is a universal favourite, but there are dozens of interesting ways to serve up fish as we show you here, and if you want chips as well, make sure you don't cheat on points tomorrow!

COD PALOOKA

8 ounces frozen cod fillets
1 ounce seasoned flour
cooking fat for frying
4 button mushrooms (peeled)
1 tomato (cut into four slices)

Separate the fillets and cut into serving portions. Coat each portion in seasoned flour and fry until golden. After turning the fish, fry mushrooms and tomatoes in the same pan and use to garnish each portion of fish. Serve hot with frozen vegetables (points extra).

Serves 2

21

HERRING CASSEROLE

1 tablespoon vegetable oil
3 ounces onion (sliced)
½ ounce plain flour
⅓ pint of white stock
8-ounce can tomatoes
2 herrings (cleaned, boned and filleted)
½ pound potatoes (peeled and cut into ⅛-inch slices)
½ teaspoon salt
Shake of pepper
1 bouquet garni

Heat the oil in a saucepan and fry the onions until golden brown. Add the flour and cook for 1 minute without browning. Gradually add the stock stirring all the time until the mixture thickens. Add the tomatoes, herrings, potatoes, salt, pepper and the bouquet garni. Place in a casserole dish and cook for 10–15 minutes or until the herrings are tender. Remove bouquet garni before serving.

Serves 2

33½

GRILLED HERRINGS WITH MUSTARD

2 fresh herrings
1 tablespoon flour
Salt and freshly ground black pepper
2 tablespoons olive oil
2 teaspoons French mustard
2 ounces breadcrumbs (freshly grated)
2 tablespoons butter (melted)

Clean and scale fresh herrings, taking care not to break the skin underneath. Cut off heads, and wash and dry fish carefully. Make three shallow incisions on sides of each fish with a sharp knife. Dip herrings in seasoned flour; brush them with olive oil and grill on a well-oiled baking sheet for 3–4 minutes on each side. Arrange herrings in a shallow ovenproof gratin dish; brush them liberally with French mustard; sprinkle with freshly grated breadcrumbs and melted butter, and put in a very hot oven (450°F/Gas 8) for 5 minutes.

Serves 2

44

FLAMED HERRINGS

2 large herrings (filleted)
2 tablespoons olive oil
2 cloves
1 teaspoon dried thyme
Seasoning
Dried thyme sprigs

Wipe the herrings dry, heat the oil in an oven-to-table pan. Into each herring insert a clove and sprinkle generously with thyme and seasoning. Place the herrings in the pan, cover and cook for 5–10 minutes or until tender, making sure they do not become dry. Sprinkle the herrings with a thick layer of thyme sprigs and bring to the table. Light the sprigs (as though they were a Christmas pudding) and when the sprigs are reduced to ashes you may add a tablespoon of hot brandy and flambé again if you like. Serve these fish either piping hot or chilled.

Serves 2

$26\frac{1}{2}$

PRAWN COCKTAIL

2 lettuce leaves
Salt and pepper
3–4 ounces peeled prawns
Pinch paprika
2 whole prawns
slices lemon

Mayonnaise Dressing:
$\frac{1}{4}$ pint mayonnaise
1 rounded teaspoon tomato purée
Dash tabasco sauce
Pinch caster sugar
Pinch cayenne pepper
Paprika pepper to decorate

Shred the lettuce leaves finely, season with salt and pepper, and arrange in two glasses. If liked, spoon on a little French dressing before serving. Mix the mayonnaise dressing ingredients together to make a fairly sharp sauce and toss the peeled prawns in it. Just before serving, spoon onto the lettuce, garnish with a pinch of paprika and a prawn and slice of lemon on the glass.
★ Without French dressing.

Serves 2

$27\frac{1}{2}$★

COD PORTUGUESE

1 ounce butter
1 medium onion (finely chopped)
2 cod steaks or cutlets (4 ounces each)
$\frac{1}{4}$ pint dry white wine
Juice half a lemon
Seasoning
2 tablespoons tomato purée
1 small tin peeled tomatoes
$\frac{1}{2}$ green pepper (blanched, seeded and chopped)
1 dessertspoon chervil or parsley (chopped)
3 stuffed olives (sliced)
1 pear (peeled, cored and thickly sliced)

Butter a medium shallow cooking pan well, scatter with chopped onion and place cod steaks in pan. Pour over the white wine and lemon juice, and season to taste. Cover with a piece of buttered greaseproof paper and poach for 10 minutes. Remove fish steaks from pan and rapidly reduce the cooking liquid. Add the tomato purée, tinned tomatoes, green pepper, chopped chervil and sliced stuffed olives. Simmer 5 minutes. Add sliced pear and simmer for a further 5 minutes. Add fish steaks to sauce and heat through gently.

Serves 2

27

BAKED FISH WITH NORMANDY SAUCE

2 fillets sole (3 ounces each)
1 tablespoon dry white wine
Salt and pepper
4 mussels (cooked)
4 button mushrooms
½ pint Normandy Sauce
Watercress

Normandy Sauce:
1 ounce butter
1 ounce flour
½ pint fish stock
1 egg yolk
Juice lemon
Salt and pepper
½ ounce butter

Fold the fillets in half and place in a buttered dish. Pour over the wine, season with salt and pepper and bake in a moderate oven, 350°F/Gas 4, for 15–20 minutes, or until the fish is opaque. Drain well, and keep the liquid. Keep the fish warm. Strain half a pint of fish stock from the fish and mussel liquor and add the mushroom trimmings, and cool. Use this to make the sauce.

Normandy Sauce:
Melt the butter, stir in the flour and cook for a few minutes. Add the fish stock slowly, stirring continuously until smooth. Bring to the boil and cook for about 4 minutes. Cool, add the egg yolk and reheat to thicken the sauce, but do not allow it to boil. Add lemon juice and seasoning and whisk in the butter.
Strain the sauce, add the mussels and halved mushrooms and heat gently. Arrange the fillets on a serving dish, pour over the sauce and garnish with watercress.

Serves 2

27

COUNTY COD

2 cod steaks
5 level tablespoons bread-crumbs
1 ounce butter
1 teaspoon parsley (finely chopped)
Large pinch mixed herbs
1 egg
Seasoning
2 rashers fat bacon

Mix together the breadcrumbs, butter, parsley and herbs, and bind with egg to a stiff mixture. Season to taste. Spread this stuffing on top of the cod steaks, placing a rasher of bacon on top of the stuffing. Well butter a shallow baking dish, put the fish in the baking dish and bake in a moderate oven, 350°F/Gas 4, for 25 minutes, or until fish is tender. Serve garnished with lemon wedges.

Serves 2

43

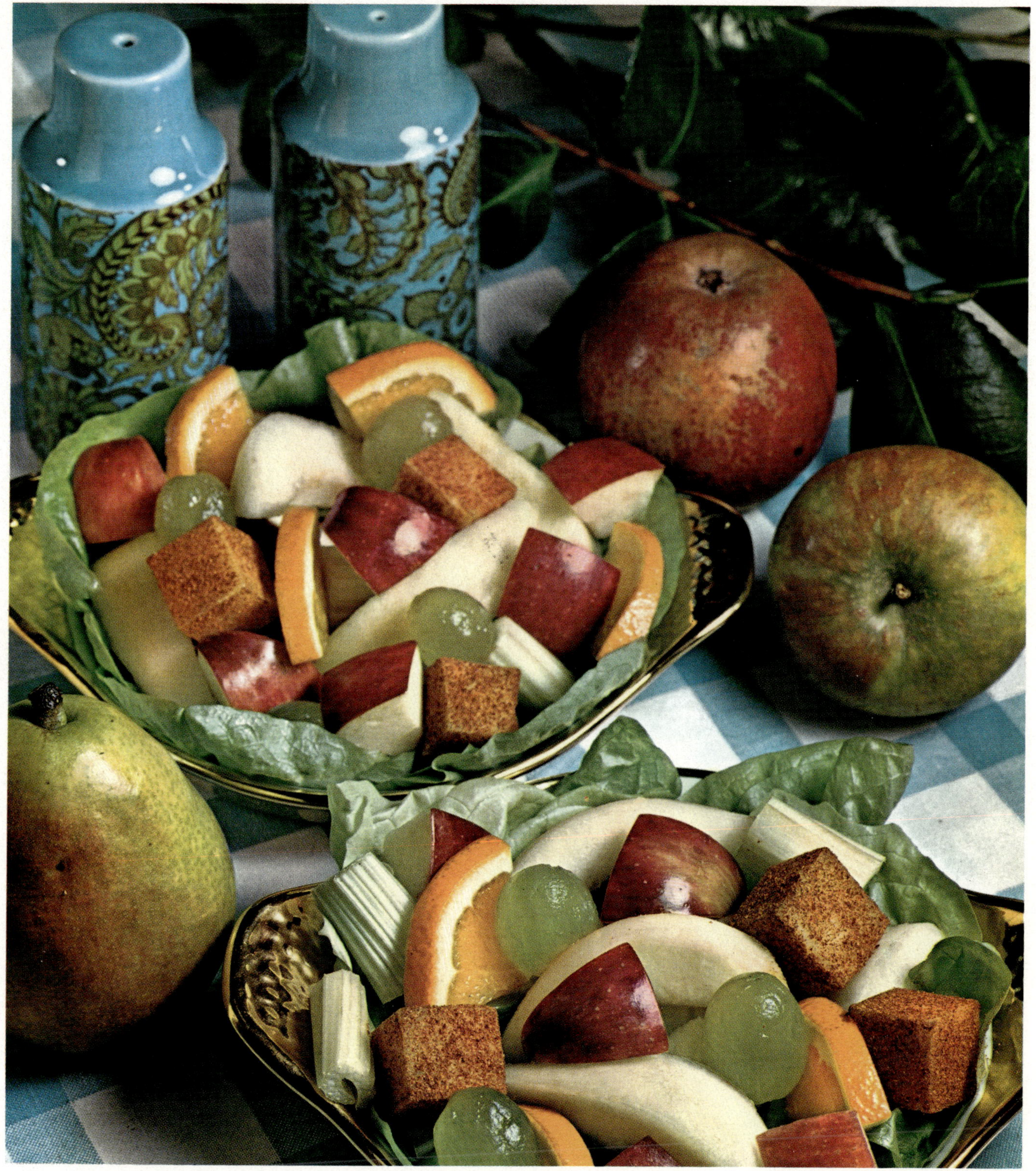

Party Snacks can look colourful, tasty and appetising with a minimum of effort.
Here is one example – Fresh Fruit Salad

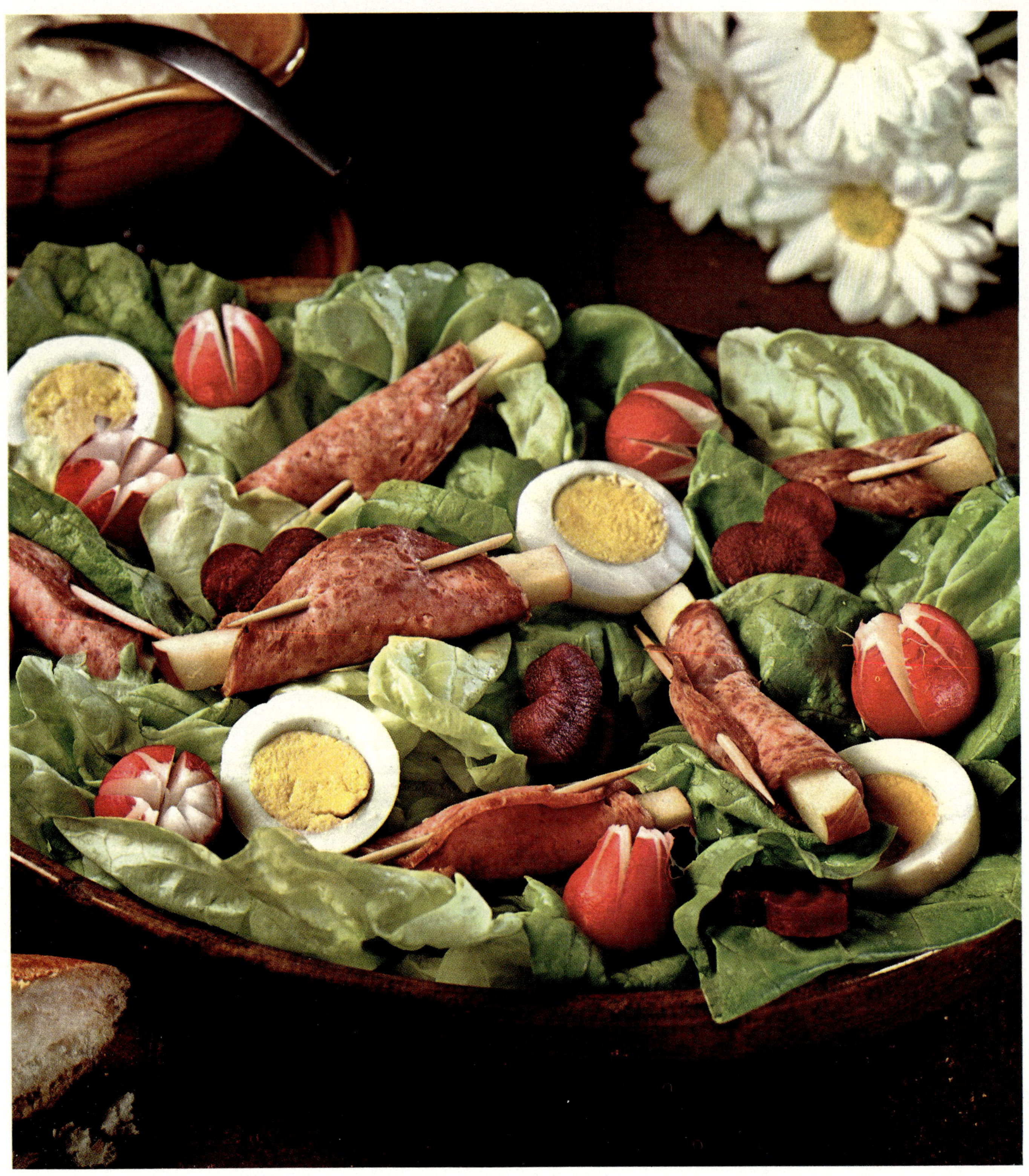

Salami Salad – another good idea for parties or social gatherings

BAKED SKATE

1 pound skate (filleted)

Sauce:
$\frac{1}{4}$ pint milk
$\frac{1}{4}$ ounce butter
Salt and pepper
Small pinch mixed dried herbs
$\frac{1}{4}$ ounce flour
1 ounce Cheddar cheese (grated)
$\frac{1}{2}$ ounce breadcrumbs (fresh)

Cut the fish into convenient sized pieces for serving. Put the milk into a pan with the butter, dried herbs and seasonings. Add the fish and cook gently till the fish is tender. Strain the liquid carefully into another saucepan and thicken with the flour mixed to a paste with a little of the fish liquor. Allow to boil for about a minute. Pour half the sauce into a shallow buttered oven dish. Add half the grated cheese. Place the fish pieces on top of the cheese. Cover with the rest of the sauce, sprinkle it with the rest of the cheese and the breadcrumbs. Bake in a moderately hot oven, 375°F/Gas 5, until the top is brown.

Serves 2

29

SOLE VERONIQUE

4 small fillets sole
$\frac{1}{8}$ pint white wine
$\frac{1}{8}$ pint fish stock
$\frac{1}{2}$ ounce butter
$\frac{1}{2}$ ounce flour
Salt and pepper
1 tablespoon cream (single)
2 ounces white grapes (skinned and with pips removed)

Season the fillets with salt and pepper to taste, then fold or roll. Place in a pan, add the wine and stock and cook very gently for about 10 minutes. Carefully remove the fish onto a hot serving dish and strain the stock. Melt the butter in a pan, do not let it brown, add the flour and mix well. Add the stock gradually, stirring continuously until the mixture boils. Remove from the heat and add the cream and the halved grapes. Reheat gently if necessary and pour over the fish.

Serves 2

23

SAVOURY HADDOCK

$\frac{1}{2}$ pound smoked haddock
2 ounces butter
Pinch cayenne pepper
2 teaspoons sweet pickle

Poach the haddock in water, remove the bones and skin, and flake the fish finely. Melt the butter in a saucepan, add the flaked haddock, a pinch of cayenne pepper and the pickle. Heat gently till very hot, and serve the mixture with triangles of toast.*

Serves 2

* 1 ounce bread (white or brown) = 3 points.

$24\frac{1}{2}$

COD CASSEROLE

2 cod steaks (4 ounces each)
1 medium onion (chopped)
1 ounce butter
level tablespoon flour
½ pint milk and water mixed in equal proportions
Seasoning
2 ounces mushrooms (sliced)
1 tablespoon parsley (chopped)
2 tomatoes (skinned and sliced)

Fry the onions in the butter until golden brown. Blend in the flour and gradually add the milk and water, stirring continuously until the mixture boils. Season to taste. Put the cod steaks in a casserole, add the mushrooms, parsley and tomatoes. Pour the sauce over the fish. Cook in a moderate oven, covered, for about 30 minutes, 350°F/Gas 4, or until the fish is cooked.

Serves 2

23

SHRIMP ENTRÉE

1 green pepper
2 tomatoes
2 small onions
3 large mushrooms
4 ounces peeled shrimps (tinned, frozen or fresh)
1 tablespoon double cream
1 cup boiled rice (4 ounces)

Cut the vegetables into strips. Sauté the peppers in a little butter, add onions, then tomatoes and sauté till tender. Add mushrooms and cook for a few minutes. Add shrimps and cream together, mixing lightly and cook for just long enough to heat the shrimps, being careful not to let the mixture boil. Serve with boiled plain rice (points extra).

Serves 2

26½

PLAICE WITH CREAMED MUSHROOM SAUCE

2 plaice (filleted)
1 ounce butter or margarine

Mushroom Sauce:
½ ounce butter
2 ounces mushrooms (thinly sliced)
3 tablespoons double cream
Juice ½ lemon
1 teaspoon parsley (chopped)
Salt and pepper

Method: Wash and trim the fish and put on the grill pan. Dot with margarine or butter. Grill under low heat for five minutes. Turn carefully, dot fish with remaining butter or margarine and grill for a further five minutes.
Sauce: Melt the butter in a small saucepan and sauté the mushrooms until tender (about 5 minutes). Add the cream, lemon juice and parsley, season to taste and reheat gently. Serve the plaice on a warmed serving dish and spoon the sauce over. Garnish with parsley and serve at once with a green vegetable.

Serves 2

32

SMOKED HADDOCK MOUSSE

Mousse:
1 ounce soft margarine
1 ounce plain flour
½ pint milk
4 fluid ounces mayonnaise or salad cream
¾ pound smoked haddock fillet (cooked and flaked)
2 hard-boiled eggs (chopped)
2–3 ounces pimento or green pepper (chopped)
4 teaspoons parsley (chopped)
½ ounce gelatine, 2½ fluid ounces fish stock } dissolved together
2½ fluid ounces double cream (whipped)

Decoration:
1 hard-boiled egg (sliced)
Parsley sprigs

Place the margarine, flour and milk into a medium-sized saucepan. Whisking all the time, over a low heat, bring to the boil and continue cooking for a further 1–2 minutes. Stir in the remaining ingredients and pour into a 1½-pint fluted mould. Place in the refrigerator to set. When set, turn out and decorate with slices of egg and sprigs of parsley.

Serves 4

78

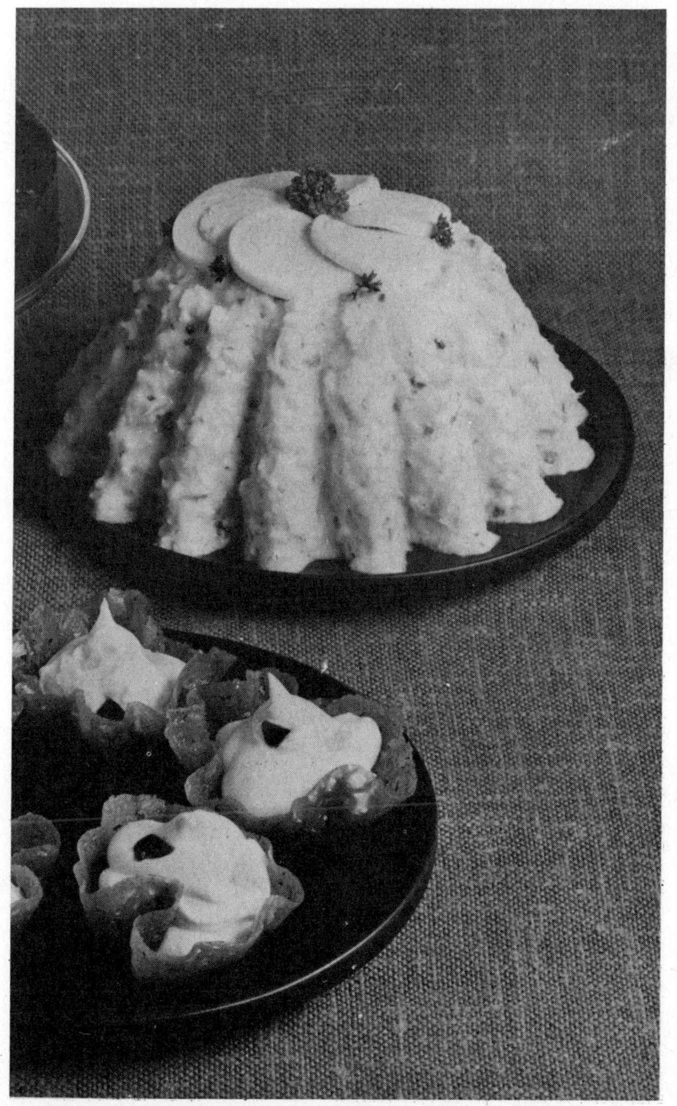

FISH CURRY

$\frac{3}{4}$ pound filleted cod
1 onion (finely chopped)
$\frac{1}{2}$ clove garlic (finely chopped)
1 tablespoon corn oil
$\frac{1}{2}$ tablespoon curry powder
1 dessertspoon tomato purée
$\frac{1}{4}$ pint cold water

Wash the fish and cut into bite-size pieces. Sauté the onion and garlic in the oil for ten minutes and stir in the curry powder. Stir well and cook gently for five minutes. Stir in the tomato purée and cook for a few minutes. Add the water gradually, stirring all the time and bring to the boil, still stirring. Put the fish into the mixture and cook very gently over a low heat for 30 minutes, or until the fish is cooked. Season to taste and serve.

Serves 2

17½

PISSALADIÈRE

1 pound onions
2 tablespoons salad oil
7-ounce tin tomatoes (drained)
1 clove garlic (crushed)*
Salt and pepper
***optional**

Dough
6 ounces self-raising flour
$\frac{1}{4}$ teaspoon salt
1½ ounces butter
$\frac{1}{8}$ pint milk
2½-ounce can anchovies
Olives for garnish

Slice the onions and cook very, very gently in the oil in a pan with a lid. The onions should be very soft and puréed and must not brown, so this will take about 40 minutes. After ten minutes, stir in the well-drained tomatoes. Add the garlic (if liked). Season.

Dough: Sift together the flour and salt. Rub in butter until mixture resembles fine breadcrumbs. Add milk enough to bind to a soft dough. Roll out into a triangle and use to line a shallow greased tin.
Spread the onion purée over the dough and arrange anchovy fillets on top in a trellis design. Bake in a hot oven, 425°F/Gas 7 for 30 minutes. Place a black olive in the centre of each trellis.

Serves 4

54

FISH CHOWDER

$\frac{1}{2}$ pound filleted cod or haddock
$\frac{1}{4}$ pint cold water
4 rashers streaky bacon (derinded)
$\frac{1}{2}$ pound potatoes (sliced thinly)
1 medium onion (sliced thinly)
Cup water
$\frac{3}{4}$ pint milk
$\frac{1}{2}$ ounce butter
Salt and pepper
Pinch paprika

Put the fish in a pan with the $\frac{1}{4}$ pint water. Bring to the boil, then simmer gently for ten minutes. Drain the fish and reserve the liquid. Remove any bones and skin from the fish and flake the fish roughly. Put the diced bacon in a pan with the potatoes and onion. Add the cup of water, cover the pan and bring to the boil. Reduce the heat and simmer for ten minutes. Add the fish and the liquid which you have reserved and simmer for a further ten minutes. Pour in the milk and bring to the boil. Just before serving add the butter and season to taste. Sprinkle with paprika.

Serves 2

60

Vegetables and Salads

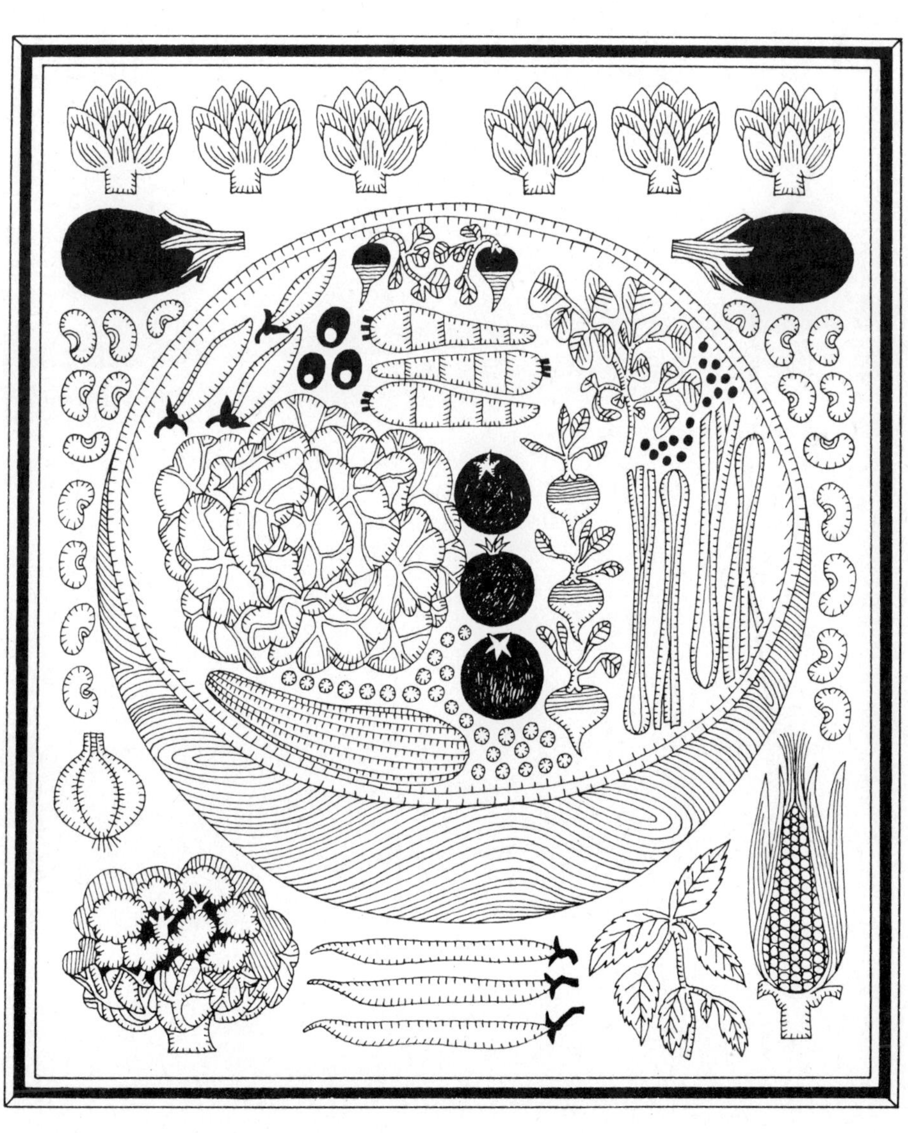

Vegetables and Salads

Obviously when you are watching your weight, salads and vegetables are an excellent choice for lunch or dinner, but there is no reason why these should be dull and 'rabbity'. There are lots of delicious ideas here, which can be enjoyed by all the family.

VEGETABLE POT-POURRI

½ small cauliflower (washed and cut into florets)
2 medium potatoes (peeled and sliced)
1 medium parsnip (peeled and sliced)
1 large onion (peeled and sliced)
Salt and pepper to taste
2 ounces Cheddar cheese (grated)
¼ pint milk
1 teaspoon Marmite

Topping:
1 ounce Cheddar cheese (grated)

Pre-heat oven to moderate, 350°F/Gas 4. Put prepared vegetables into a greased heatproof dish in alternate layers. Sprinkle each layer with cheese and season with salt and pepper. Heat milk and add Marmite. Pour over vegetables and sprinkle top heavily with cheese. Cover and cook in centre of oven for about 1 hour. Serve immediately.

Serves 2

35

VEGETABLE HOT POT

½ pound green cabbage
½ pound potatoes (peeled)
1 large onion (sliced)
2 ounces butter
Salt and pepper
Large pinch mixed herbs

Slice cabbage and cook in boiling water, salted, for 10 minutes. Drain. Cut potatoes into ¼-inch slices and cook in boiling salted water for 5–7 minutes. Drain. Fry onions in 1 ounce butter until tender but not browned. Use a little of the remaining butter to butter an ovenproof casserole. Arrange cabbage, onion and potatoes in layers with seasonings and herbs in casserole, finishing with potato. Dot with remaining butter and brown in hot oven (425°F/Gas 7) for 30 minutes.

Serves 2

30

CARROTS AND CELERY IN CIDER

½ pint dry cider
½ pound carrots
½ head celery (4 large sticks)
Salt and pepper
Parsley (chopped)

Bring the cider to boiling point. Prepare the vegetables and cut into 2-inch strips. The outside stalks of the celery should be used. Add the carrots to the cider and boil gently for 15 minutes. Add the celery with the seasonings and cook for a further 30 minutes. Retaining the liquid, drain the vegetables and keep hot. Boil the cider quickly until reduced to about 2 tablespoons. Pour over the vegetables, sprinkle with parsley and serve hot.

Serves 2

7

RATATOUILLE

1 large onion (sliced thinly)
1 ounce butter
1 tablespoon corn oil
1 aubergine (sliced)
$\frac{1}{2}$ pound marrow (sliced)
$\frac{1}{2}$ large green pepper (deseeded and chopped)
1 level tablespoon chopped parsley
$\frac{1}{2}$ pound tomatoes (skinned and chopped)
Salt

Fry the onion in the oil and butter in a saucepan for about five minutes. Add the aubergine and marrow, and tomatoes and pepper. Mix gently, cover pan and simmer gently for about 1 hour.

Serves 2

20

CAULIFLOWER WITH CHEESE

1 medium-sized cauliflower
2 ounces butter
1 level dessertspoon onion (finely grated)
4 ounces Cheddar cheese (grated)

Cook the cauliflower in boiling salted water until tender, then drain and divide into florets. Fry the onion in the butter until soft but not brown, add the cauliflower and fry gently, turning frequently until golden. Transfer to a warm serving dish, sprinkle with cheese and brown quickly under a hot grill.

Serves 2

44

STUFFED MARROW

1 small marrow
2 ounces onion (chopped)
Cup of stock
Teaspoon tomato purée
6 ounces cooked meat (minced)
$\frac{1}{2}$ egg
2 tablespoons breadcrumbs
Salt and pepper

Wash the outside of the marrow and cut it in half lengthways. Place in a pan of boiling salted water and simmer for ten minutes. Chop the onion. Add the tomato purée to the stock. Place in a pan with the onions and simmer until most of the stock has been absorbed. Beat the egg and mix with the minced cooked meat breadcrumbs and onions. Drain. Fill the cavity with the meat mixture. Bake in a baking tin with a small amount of stock for 45 minutes at 375°F/Gas 5.

Serves 2

28

PEAR AND CHEESE SALAD

1 pear (peeled, cored and chopped)
1 small banana (peeled and sliced)
1 fluid ounce lemon juice
3 ounces Cheddar cheese (diced)
1½ ounces Danish blue cheese (diced)
4 radishes (washed)

Toss the pears and bananas in the lemon juice. Mix with all the remaining ingredients. Arrange lettuce round the edge of a serving bowl. Pour some vinegar or lemon juice over the salad mixture if liked, and pile into the centre of the lettuce and serve.

Serves 2

25

BEEF AND APPLE SALAD

½ pound cold lean roast beef (diced)
8 radishes (washed, topped and tailed and sliced)
1 apple (cored and sliced)
2 sticks celery (diced)
4 tablespoons French dressing

Mix all the prepared meat and vegetables together in a bowl. Pour over about 4 tablespoons of French dressing made according to taste. Arrange in a serving dish and sprinkle with chopped parsley.

Serves 2

36½

APPLE FRANKFURTER SALAD

Lettuce (6 leaves)
2 large cooked frankfurters (sliced)
2 tomatoes (quartered)
1 eating apple (cored and diced)
1 tablespoon Mayonnaise
Seasoning
2 rashers cooked, lean bacon (diced)
Parsley

Arrange a bed of lettuce in a salad bowl. Arrange a border of sliced frankfurter and quartered tomatoes. Mix together apple, mayonnaise and seasoning and pile in the centre of the salad. Sprinkle with diced, cooked bacon. Garnish with parsley.

Serves 2

19

LAMB SALAD AMONDINE

$\frac{1}{2}$ pound cooked shoulder or leg lamb (lean)
1 stick celery (chopped)
1 ounce flaked almonds
$\frac{1}{2}$ small red pepper (deseeded and chopped)
2 tablespoons mayonnaise
1 small pinch celery salt
Lettuce (6 leaves)

Cut the lamb into small pieces. Add celery, almonds and pepper. Mix together celery salt and mayonnaise and toss lamb and vegetables in the mixture and chill. Place lettuce leaves on serving dish and pile the lamb salad onto the lettuce leaves. Serve immediately.

Serves 2

41

CRUNCHY MIXED SALAD

8 ounces white cabbage
a few black grapes (halved and de-seeded)
a few green grapes (halved and de-seeded)
6 walnut halves
8 pineapple chunks (drained)
Small lettuce heart (washed)
$\frac{1}{2}$ red skinned apple
lemon juice

Dressing:
2 tablespoons olive oil
1 tablespoon wine vinegar
1 level tablespoon sugar
Salt
Pepper

Method: Place the shredded cabbage in very cold water to crisp. Prepare the other ingredients. Line a suitable bowl with lettuce leaves and pile the drained white cabbage in the centre. Cut the apple half, remove the core, and cut the flesh into pieces, dip in lemon juice and arrange on a bed of lettuce. Scatter on other ingredients. Mix all the ingredients for the dressing and serve separately.

Serves 2

33

PRUNE STUFFED TOMATOES

4 large firm tomatoes
$1\frac{1}{2}$ ounces butter
3 tablespoons cream cheese (low fat)
6 prunes (cooked)

To serve: Lettuce (4-5 leaves)

Cut a circle about $1\frac{1}{4}$ inches across from the top of each tomato. Scoop out inside with a teaspoon and turn upside down on kitchen paper to drain. Cream butter and beat in cream cheese. Stone and chop all the prunes except for one. Add the chopped prunes, 1 tablespoon of prune syrup to butter and cheese mixture. Mix well and use to fill centres of tomatoes. Divide the remaining prune into quarters and use one quarter to top each of the tomatoes. Serve with lettuce.

Serves 4

35

YOGURT SALAD DRESSING

1 carton natural yogurt (unsweetened)
2 tablespoons single cream or top of the bottle
3 teaspoons lemon juice
1 level teaspoon caster sugar
$\frac{1}{4}$ teaspoon salt
Pinch pepper

Put the yogurt in a bowl and beat in the cream, lemon juice and sugar. Season to taste. This is best left in the fridge or cool larder for $\frac{1}{2}$–1 hour before using.

7$\frac{1}{2}$

Sweets

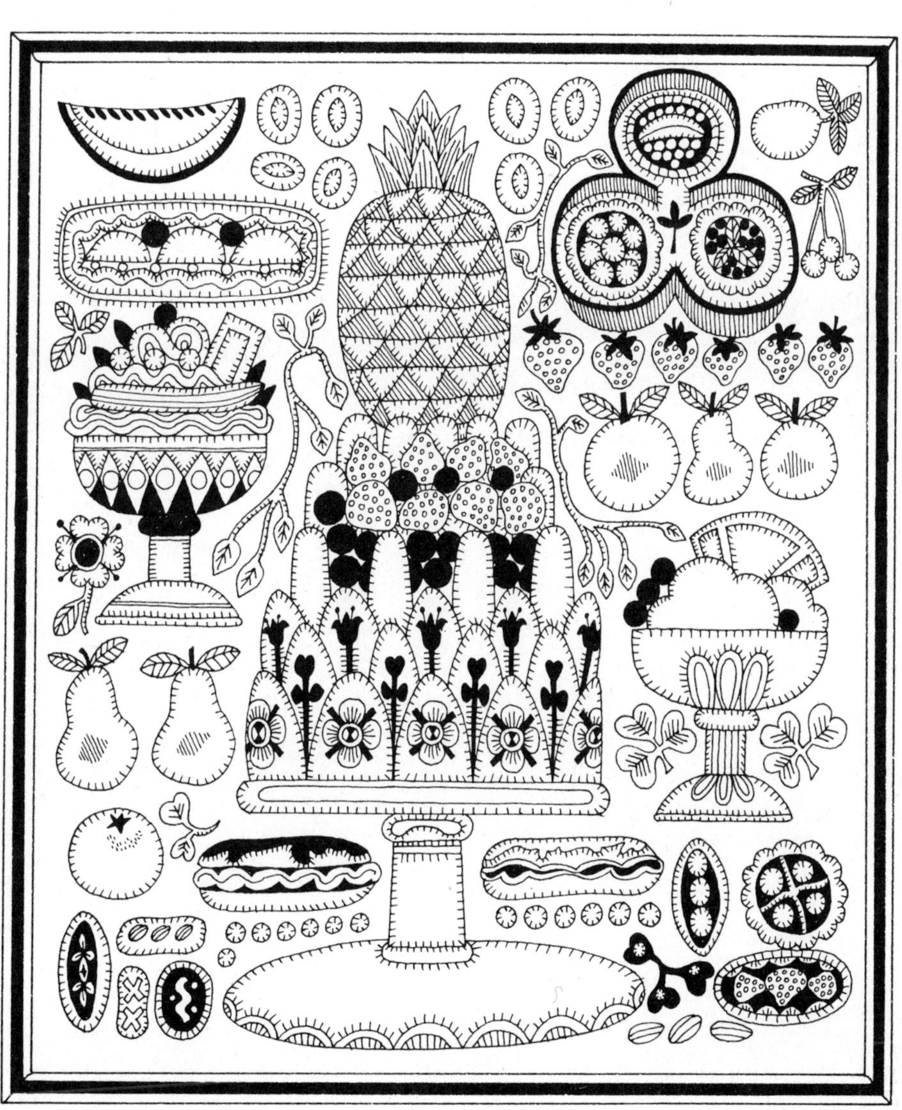

If you have a sweet tooth—and who hasn't?—you won't be able to resist some of the luscious sweets we have for you here. The children will like the ice cream recipes while Dad will probably prefer some of the more substantial sweets, but whichever recipes you try, you will find them delicious.

SICILIAN CASSATA

$\frac{1}{2}$ pint milk
3 large eggs
4 ounces caster sugar
1 ounce soft margarine
4 tablespoons cream (double or single)
2 ounces plain chocolate (melted over hot water)
1$\frac{1}{2}$ ounces mixed sultanas and raisins
2 ounces chopped fruits (apricots, cherries, etc.)
1 ounce angelica (chopped)
2 teaspoons orange curaçao (optional)
Orange food colouring

Place milk, eggs and sugar in a double saucepan over a medium heat and stir until thick (about 5 minutes). Remove from heat and cool. Add margarine and cream, beating thoroughly. Divide mixture in half. To one half add the melted chocolate, to the other add the fruits, curaçao and colouring. Place chocolate ice cream in a 1-pound loaf tin, leave 'fruity' ice cream in basin and place both in the freezing compartment set at the coldest setting. When partially set (1–1$\frac{1}{2}$ hours) stir the ice creams vigorously with a fork. Return to freezer. When on point of setting, spread chocolate ice cream round the sides and bottom of the loaf tin and fill the middle with 'fruity' ice cream, pressing down firmly. Re-freeze for about 1 hour until firm. Serve with fresh fruit.

Serves 6

81

PEAR AND LEMON DESSERT

4 pears (peeled, halved and cored)
2 tablespoons lemon juice
Rind and juice 1 lemon
2 ounces caster sugar
$\frac{1}{2}$ pint water
$\frac{1}{4}$ ounce gelatine dissolved in 1 tablespoon hot water
8 maraschino cherries (dried)
Little yellow colouring

To decorate:
Crystallized lemon slices

Marinate the pear halves in the lemon juice to prevent discolouration. Stand the lemon rind, juice and sugar in the water for an hour, then place in a pan and bring to the boil. Simmer for 5 minutes, add the colouring and cool. Stir in the gelatine and allow to go cold. Place a cherry in each pear half and arrange four halves around the outside of each sundae glass. When the jelly is nearly set, fill the glasses up. When firm, decorate the top with crystallized lemon slices.

Serves 4

20

TASMAN PUDDING

Batter mixture:
2 ounces plain flour
Small pinch salt
$\frac{1}{2}$ egg
$\frac{1}{4}$ pint milk

Filling:
$\frac{1}{2}$ pound apples (peeled and sliced)
1 ounce sultanas
Juice of $\frac{1}{2}$ small lemon
$\frac{1}{2}$ tablespoon caster sugar
$\frac{1}{2}$ tablespoon clear honey
$\frac{1}{2}$ ounce butter

Sieve the flour and salt into a basin. Make a well in the middle. Break the egg into a cup and pour half into the well. Add about a quarter of the milk and carefully blend in the flour. Then beat really hard with a wooden spoon until the mixture is smooth. Allow to stand for half an hour. Then slowly add the remaining milk, beating all the time. Let the batter stand for at least half an hour before using.
Meanwhile, grease the bottom and sides of an ovenproof dish and arrange the apple slices in the bottom. Sprinkle on the sultanas, the lemon juice, sugar and honey. Place in a hot oven 425°F/Gas 7 for 10 minutes. Give the batter another beating, then pour it over the fruit. Put the dish back into the oven and cook for a further 40 minutes, reducing heat to 350°F/Gas 4 after 15 minutes to prevent burning. Serve hot with custard.

Serves 4

28

QUEENSLAND PUDDING

Topping:
1 ounce butter
1 ounce soft brown sugar
$\frac{1}{2}$ tin mandarin oranges
2 ounces sultanas

Sponge:
2 ounces butter
2 ounces caster sugar
1 egg
3 ounces self-raising flour

First make the topping. Melt the butter slowly in a small saucepan with the brown sugar and $\frac{1}{2}$ tablespoon mandarin syrup. Pour into a 6-inch cake tin. Sprinkle on the sultanas and orange segments.
Now make the sponge: Cream the butter and sugar until light and fluffy. Beat in the egg and fold in the flour. Spoon on top of the sultanas and mandarins, and smooth carefully. Bake at 400°F/Gas 6 for about 25 minutes or until the sponge is firm. Turn out and serve hot with custard or cream if desired.

Serves 4

66

ORANGE CHEESE CAKE

For the base:
1½ ounces semi-sweet biscuits
1 tablespoon caster sugar
1 ounce margarine

For the cake:
9 ounces cream cheese
3 tablespoons orange squash
1 standard egg
1 level dessertspoon flour
1 level dessertspoon caster sugar

For decoration:
1 large orange
6 tablespoons cold water
3 tablespoons orange squash
2 level teaspoons arrowroot

Crush biscuits powder fine and mix with the caster sugar. Melt margarine and brush the sides and base of a 6-inch loose-based tin with margarine. Mix remaining margarine into biscuits. Press into base of tin. Blend cream cheese until smooth, gradually adding the orange squash. Separate egg and mix the flour and the caster sugar with the yolk. Add to cheese mixture. Beat egg white until stiff, add cheese mixture and fold together carefully. Pour into prepared tin. Bake at 325°F/Gas 3 for 40–45 minutes. Allow to cool in tin. Remove cheese cake from tin and place on a plate, keeping metal base in position. Remove peel from orange and cut into thin slices. Place on top, overlapping each slice to form a circle. Mix orange squash with arrowroot, bring water to boil and add arrowroot, return to boil and stir until glaze is clear and thickened. Cool slightly and pour over top and sides to glaze. Chill before serving.

Serves 6

107

APPLE AND LEMON RING

1 pint milk
4 ounces rice
1 cooking apple (peeled, cored and diced)
2 ounces sugar
½ pint double cream (whipped)
3 tablespoons lemon curd
1 tablespoon lemon juice
Little water
3 dessert apples (peeled, cored and sliced)
Grated chocolate

Bring milk to boil and add rice. Stir until milk boils again. Add diced apple. Cover and simmer until rice is thick and creamy. Stir in sugar and cool. Add double cream, stirring well. Turn into a ring mould and place in refrigerator for at least an hour. Heat lemon curd, lemon juice and water until boiling. Add apple slices and keep simmering until apple slices are tender (5–6 minutes). Allow to cool. When required turn out rice mould, fill centre with apple and lemon curd mixture and arrange remainder round base of mould. Sprinkle with grated chocolate.

Serves 4

122

PEACH AND GINGER CRUNCH

1 tablespoon custard powder
2 tablespoons sugar
$\frac{1}{2}$ pint milk
Rind and juice of 1 small lemon
3 peaches (peeled, stoned and diced)
12 ginger biscuits (crushed finely)

Make up the custard blend in the usual way by mixing the custard powder with the sugar and a little of the measured milk. Heat the rest of the milk until steaming, pour over the custard powder, stirring. Return to the saucepan and bring to the boil. Boil for a few minutes, then remove from the heat. Add the lemon rind and juice, fold in the diced peaches and allow the mixture to cool. When cold, spoon some of the custard mixture into two individual dishes. Sprinkle over a layer of crushed ginger biscuits. Repeat these layers until the dishes are full. Chill before serving.

Serves 4

33

FLOATING ISLANDS

$\frac{1}{2}$ packet lime flavoured jelly
1 pint freshly made custard (sweetened)
1 egg white
1 ounce caster sugar

Pour the custard into a serving dish and leave until completely cold. Meanwhile make up the jelly as directed on the packet with 3 tablespoons boiling water only. Cool until just setting. Make a stiff meringue by whipping the egg white and the caster sugar, then gradually fold in the jelly. Pile, in dessertspoons, on top of the custard and chill before serving.

Serves 4

40

FOAM PUDDING

1 ounce butter
$2\frac{1}{2}$ tablespoons golden syrup
1 egg
1 small lemon
1 level tablespoon self-raising flour
$\frac{1}{2}$ teacup milk

Beat the butter with the syrup and egg yolk. Stir in the grated rind and juice of the lemon, flour and half the milk. Beat the egg white until stiff enough to hold peaks then fold into the mixture and add the rest of the milk. Grease a small ovenproof dish and pour the mixture in. Stand in a baking tin with water coming half way up the side of the baking dish and bake at 350°F/Gas 4 for about 40 minutes.

Serves 2

26

BAKED PEACHES

2 peaches
2 teaspoons raspberry jam
2 tablespoons boiling water
$\frac{1}{2}$ dessertspoon lemon juice
1 tablespoon sugar (sweetener)

Place the peaches in a bowl, cover with boiling water and leave for just half a minute. Remove from the water and remove the skin from the peaches. Halve the peaches, remove the stone and place $\frac{1}{2}$ teaspoon jam in each cavity. Place the peaches in a fireproof oven dish, with the jam side uppermost. Add the sugar and lemon juice to the 2 tablespoons boiling water and pour this round the peaches. Cover closely and bake in a slow oven, 325°F/Gas 3 for 15–20 minutes.

Serves 2

9

TIGER RING

3 ounces margarine
3 ounces caster sugar
2 small eggs
3 ounces self-raising flour
1 ounce cocoa powder
Pinch salt
Dessertspoon hot water

Cream the margarine and caster sugar together; gradually beat in the eggs and then fold in the flour and salt. Divide the mixture in half. Mix the cocoa and water together and stir this into half the cake mixture. Put a layer of the chocolate mixture, then a layer of the plain mixture into a greased bowl and continue to alternate the layers until all the mixture is used. Cover with doubled greaseproof paper or foil and tie tightly and steam for 1 hour. Turn out and serve with custard or chocolate sauce.

Serves 4

65

MOCHA SUNDAE

1 family block coffee ice cream
Chopped nuts
Whipped cream

Chocolate sauce:
4 tablespoons clear honey
4 ounces plain chocolate (roughly broken into pieces)

Make the sauce by warming the honey until hot but not boiling. Stir in the chocolate until dissolved. Allow to cool until lukewarm. Fill up sundae glasses with alternate layers of ice cream, chocolate sauce and chopped nuts. Finish with a scoop of ice cream. Top with whipped cream or flaked chocolate.

Serves 4

69

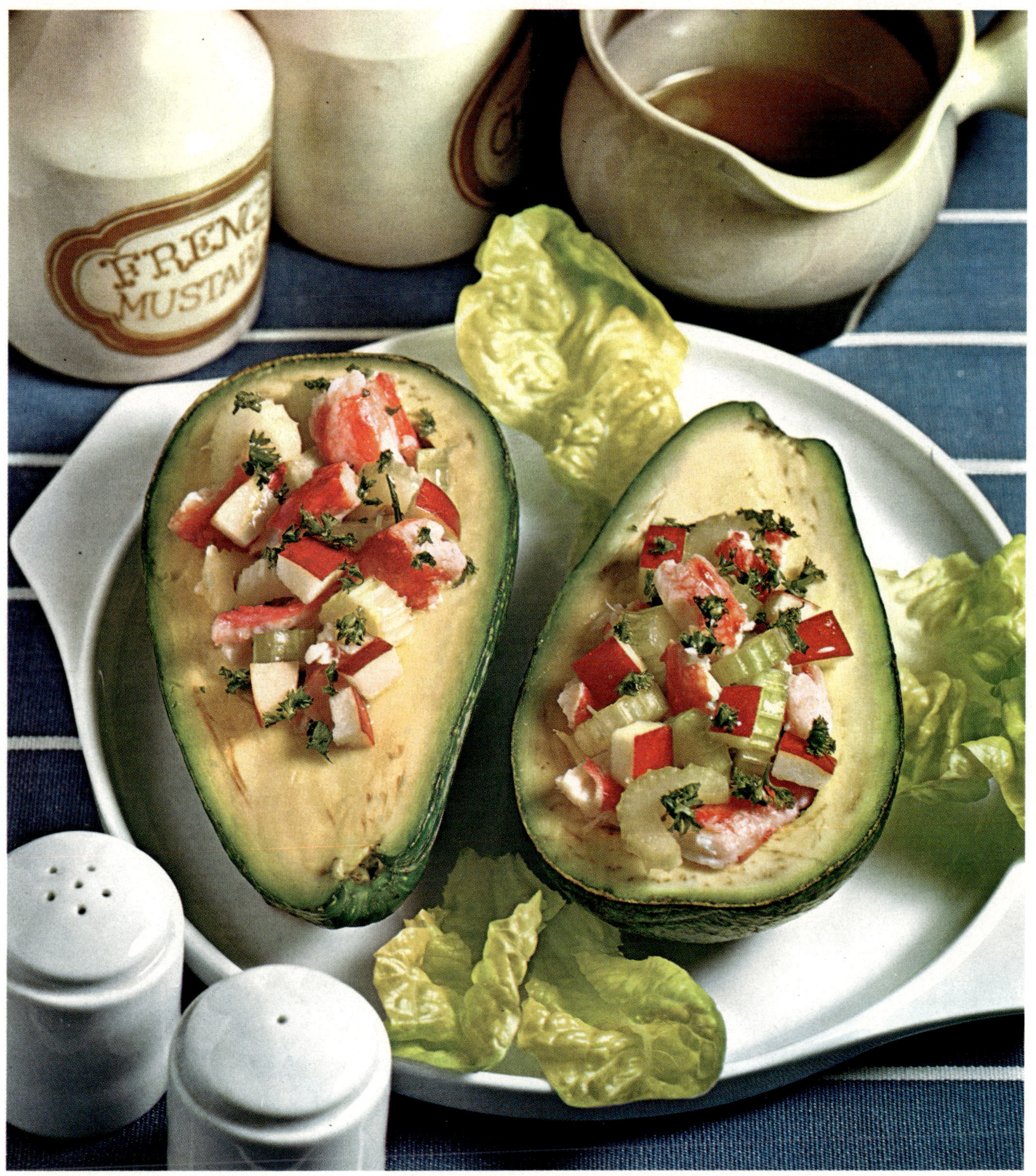

A delicious starter – avocados sprinkled with apple, celery and prawns

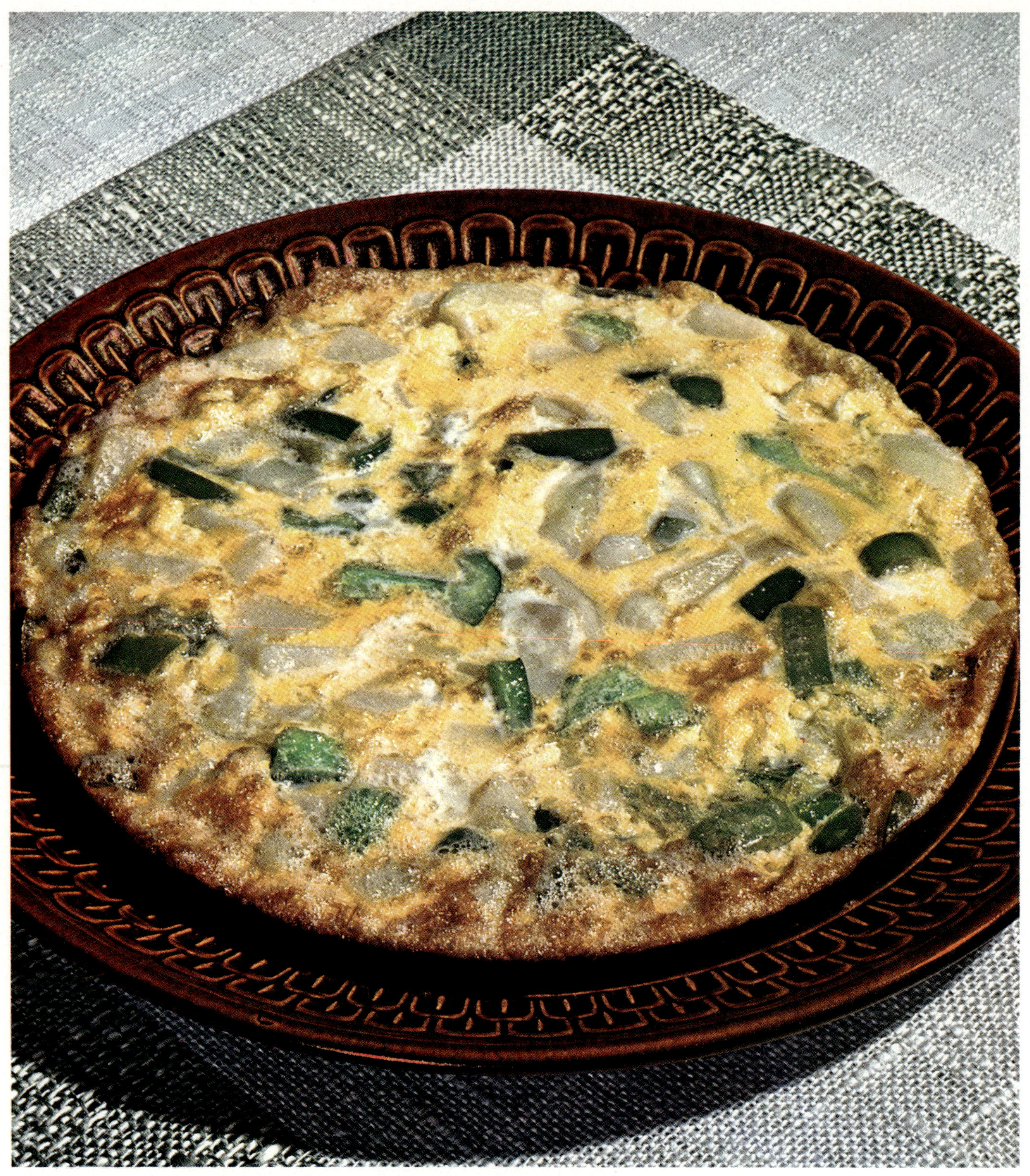

A tasty lunch-time omelette – add cooked potato, onion and green pepper when eggs are almost cooked. (Other omelette ideas on pages 20 and 23)

ALMOND CRUST PEARS

2 even-size ripe pears
Juice of $\frac{1}{2}$ lemon
2 tablespoons apricot jam (sieved and melted)
2 ounces toasted chopped almonds
Tinned peach slices (optional)

Peel the pears carefully, leaving the stalks intact. Brush the pears with lemon juice, and then with the prepared apricot jam. Coat evenly with the chopped toasted almonds. Arrange on a serving plate and garnish, if liked, with peach slices.

20

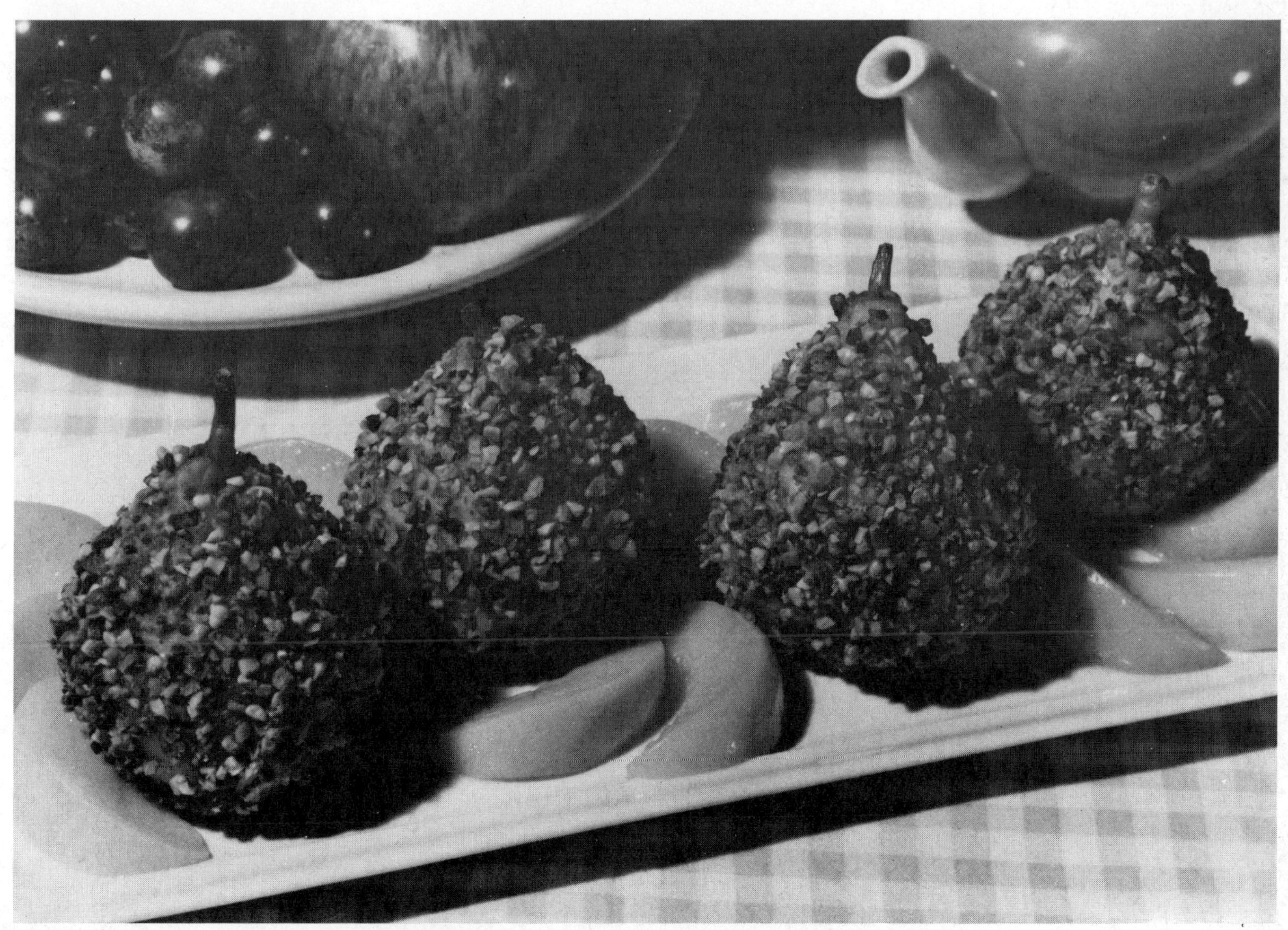

COFFEE CLOUD

½ ounce envelope of gelatine
2 tablespoons cold water
4 tablespoons boiling water
3 level dessertspoons granulated sugar
2 tablespoons coffee essence
½ pint cold milk
2 egg whites

Soften gelatine for 5 minutes in cold water. Add boiling water and sugar and stir until dissolved. Pour in coffee essence and milk, then leave the mixture in a cold place until just beginning to thicken. Whisk until frothy then slowly whisk in egg whites, which have been beaten until stiff and peaky. When the mixture is smooth, pour into a 1½–2-pint fancy mould which has been rinsed out with cold water. Chill overnight. Turn out and serve decorated with grated chocolate and whipped cream.

Serves 4

18

APPLE CRISP

3 tart eating apples
1 tablespoon lemon juice
3 level tablespoons flour
3 level tablespoons brown sugar
¼ teaspoon ground cinnamon
2 ounces butter

To decorate:
Apple skin
Glacé cherry

Peel, core and slice the apple and place the slices in a well-buttered baking dish. Sprinkle with lemon juice. Mix the flour, brown sugar, cinnamon and butter with a fork until the mixture is crumbly. Sprinkle over the apples and bake in the oven at 350°F/Gas 4 for 35 minutes, or until apples are tender.

Serves 2

34

PINEAPPLE POLL

½ ounce butter
1 ounce soft brown sugar
Juice 1 orange
2 pineapple rings
1 tablespoon brandy
½ family block Cornish ice cream

Melt the butter in a small saucepan, stir in the sugar and the orange juice, and heat very gently until the sugar is dissolved. Poach the pineapple rings in this syrup for five minutes. Drain and place on a warm serving dish. Reduce the syrup slightly until it thickens. Divide the ice cream into two and place half on each of the pineapple rings. Add the brandy to the syrup and pour over the pineapple and ice cream. Serve immediately.

Serves 2

24½

SPICY FANTASY

6 ounces flan pastry
1 pound rhubarb
4 fluid ounces milk
2 ounces granulated sugar
¾ teaspoon ground ginger
¼ teaspoon ground nutmeg
1 packet Dream Topping

Line a flan tin with the pastry. Cut the rhubarb into small pieces and arrange in the flan case. Sprinkle with the sugar, ½ teaspoon ground ginger and the ground nutmeg. Bake in a hot oven 450°F/Gas 8 for 10 minutes, and then reduce the oven heat to 350°F/Gas 4 for a further 30 minutes. Make up the Dream Topping as directed on the packet and whisk in ¼ teaspoon ground ginger. Decorate the flan with this.

Serves 4

58

CHOCOLATE MOUSSE

2 eggs
2 ounces plain chocolate
2 teaspoons water

Melt the chocolate with the water in a basin over hot water. Stir until smooth. Separate eggs. Beat yolks into melted chocolate. Leave until cool. Whisk the egg whites stiffly and fold lightly into the chocolate mixture. Make sure they are perfectly blended. Pour into individual serving dishes and leave to set. Serve with whipped cream or decorated with grated chocolate.
You can vary this recipe by adding the grated rind of 1 orange with the egg yolk and using orange juice instead of water.

Serves 2

19½

ORANGE AND LEMON SHIMMER

1 packet lemon jelly
3 oranges
Angelica for decoration

Make up the jelly as directed on the packet. Set about half an inch of jelly in the base of a 1-pint jelly mould. Peel and divide the oranges into segments, removing the pith and seeds. Arrange the orange segments on top of the set jelly. Pour over another layer of liquid jelly, allow to set, then repeat the layer of orange segments. Repeat this process until the mould is full, reserving a few orange segments for decoration. Allow jelly to set completely in a cool place. Turn out when set and decorate with orange segments and pieces of angelica.

Serves 4

19½

STRAWBERRY PETAL TARTLETS

6 ounces plain flour
½ teaspoon salt
3 ounces butter
2 ounces sugar
1 egg yolk
2 teaspoons water

Filling:
¼ pint double cream
½ pound strawberries

You will also need 6 saucers

Sift flour and salt into a bowl. Rub in butter until mixture resembles fine breadcrumbs, then add sugar. Blend egg and water, add to flour and bind together to form a stiff dough. Leave to rest for 10 minutes in a cool place. Roll out pastry thinly and cut out 36 circles with a 2-inch plain butter. Place 5 circles, slightly overlapping, round edges of 6 saucers. Dampen each overlapping edge and centre edges with a little water. Cover centre of saucers with remaining 6 pastry circles. Push down firmly and prick well. Bake in a moderate oven, 375°F/Gas 5, for 25 minutes until golden brown. Remove carefully and cool.

Whip cream until just stiff. Cut strawberries in half, keeping 6 whole ones for decoration, and sweeten with a little sugar if necessary. Spoon cream in centre of each tart. Place cut strawberries round outside of cream with points facing outwards. Place the whole strawberries in centre of cream.

Serves 6

130½

STUFFED BAKED PEARS

2 fresh pears (peeled, cored and halved)
Juice of 1 lemon

Filling:
Chopped ginger with syrup (*or* raisins and blanched almonds)

Apricot Glaze:
2 tablespoons apricot jam
1 tablespoon water

Soak pear halves with lemon juice, place in a baking dish and half fill the baking dish with water. Mix the filling of your choice, and spoon it into the scooped-out centre of each pear half, cover with buttered greaseproof paper or foil and bake in a moderate oven 375°F/Gas 5 for 20 minutes, or until pears are tender. Drain and place on a serving dish. Brush with apricot glaze, made by boiling jam and water together for 3 minutes and then sieving before use. Decorate the pear halves before serving with cherries and sprigs of mint.

Serves 2

10

Instant Food

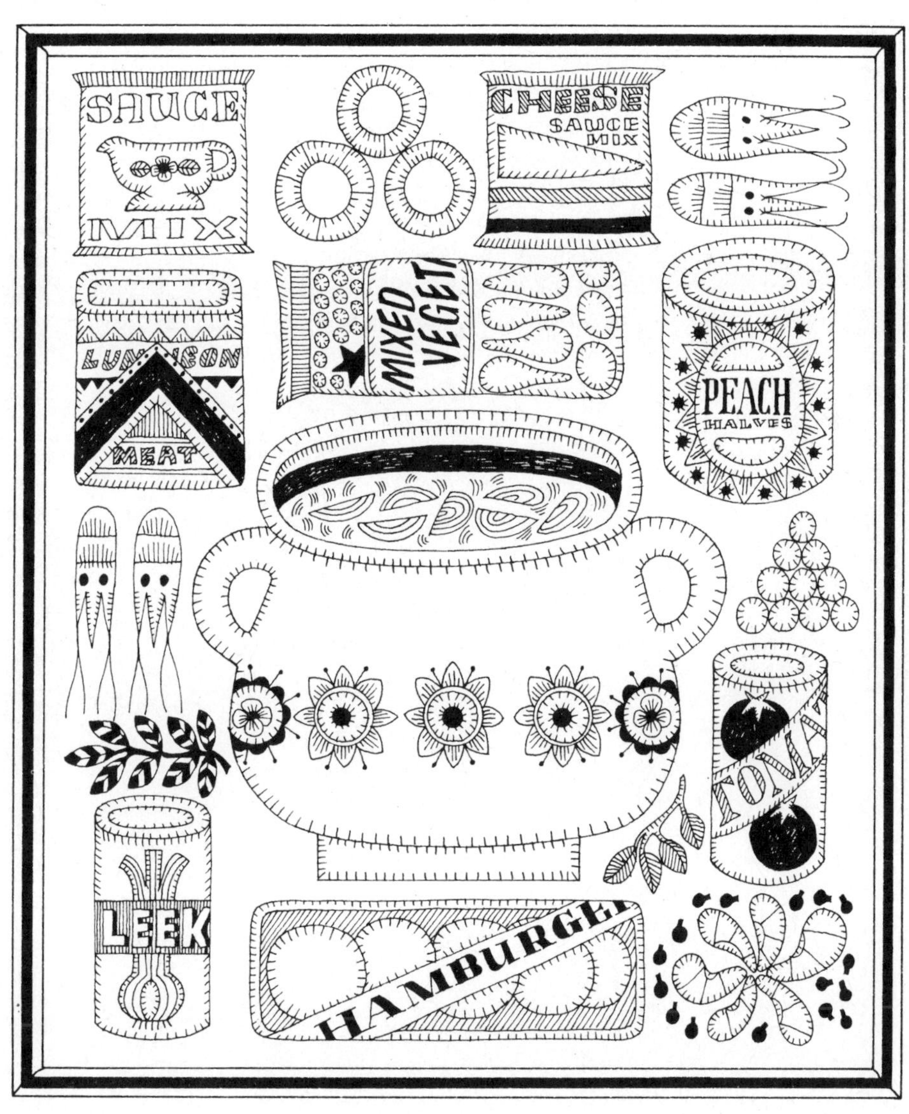

Instant Food

Some housewives feel they have cheated if they serve a curry with no more effort than that required for snipping off the packet corner with a pair of scissors! Others blush when serving frozen vegetables, apologise for frozen chips, and feel guilty if they put on the table a ready-made tinned dessert. What nonsense!

Dehydrated, frozen and tinned foods are 'instant' cookery and there to be used when you want 'instant' meals.

SPICY HAM AND PEACH

1 7-ounce can luncheon meat
1 8-ounce can sliced peaches

Sauce:
¼ pint tomato ketchup
1 tablespoon Worcestershire sauce
2 tablespoons peach syrup from can
Juice half a lemon
Dash tabasco sauce
Pinch cinnamon

Cut the meat into four slices and arrange in a shallow fireproof dish with the peach slices in between. Mix all the sauce ingredients together and pour over the meat. Heat for 15 minutes at 375°F/Gas 5 and serve.

Serves 2

40

PORCUPINES OR BEEF BALLS

1 large packet frozen beefburgers (4)
2 cups tomato juice
5 whole cloves
1 tablespoon Worcestershire sauce
1 tablespoon onion (chopped)
1 tablespoon green pepper (finely chopped)

Defrost beefburgers according to instructions. Heat tomato juice, cloves and Worcestershire sauce. Mix beefburgers, chopped onion, chopped green pepper, and form into balls about 1½ inches diameter. Remove cloves from tomato sauce, put in the meat balls, cover and simmer 45–50 minutes.

Serves 2

30

QUICK GOULASH

1 10½-ounce can condensed tomato soup
1 15½-ounce can stewed steak with onions
½ meat cube (dissolved in a little water)
½ level teaspoon paprika pepper
½ teaspoon cornflour
Glass dry red wine
Dash Worcestershire sauce
Squeeze of lemon juice
Black pepper and garlic salt to taste
½ small carton soured cream

Empty the soup into a saucepan and add the meat. Stir in the meat cube and the paprika pepper. Mix the cornflour with the red wine and add this to the saucepan. Bring to the boil and add the Worcestershire sauce, lemon juice, black pepper and garlic salt to taste. When boiling, reduce heat and stir in the soured cream. Serve with rice or noodles (*see* appendix for points).

Serves 2

50

Why not use them with pride and serve them with a flourish? Practise your own individual tricks when 'dressing up' instant dishes; for example, you can garnish tinned or packet soup with frankfurter slices, chopped cooked bacon, a slice of lemon, grated cheese, salted whipped cream, chopped mint or parsley, chopped egg or chives, or toasted almond slivers.

PRAWNS AND BACON

1 4-ounce tin (or frozen) prawns (chopped finely)
4 rashers lean bacon
1 egg
1 tablespoon corn oil
1 dessertspoon onion (chopped)
1 packet mushroom sauce
½ pint milk
1 level teaspoon cornflour

Spread the prawns onto the bacon rashers and roll up tightly. If necessary secure with a cocktail stick. Coat with cornflour and dip in the beaten egg. Heat the corn oil and fry the bacon rolls until brown, turning several times to make sure they brown evenly. Keep warm on a hot dish.
Gently fry the onion in the remaining oil, and add the onion to the made-up mushroom sauce. Pour over the bacon rolls and serve (removing cocktail sticks before doing so).

Serves 2

43

SAVOURY SUPPER

1 packet savoury white sauce
½ pint milk
3 ounces Cheddar cheese (grated)
2 hard-boiled eggs
1 small packet frozen mixed vegetables
4 rashers bacon (cut into pieces)

Make up the white sauce as instructed on the packet. Stir in 2 ounces of cheese. Pour enough of the sauce into the bottom of a small oven dish to cover the bottom. Arrange slices of hard-boiled egg, mixed vegetables and bacon in layers and then pour the remaining sauce over. Sprinkle with the rest of the cheese and brown in a hot oven, 425°F/Gas 7, for about 10 minutes.

Serves 2

60

FARMHOUSE SUPPER

1 small (1 pound) cauliflower (cooked)
2 carrots (tinned, sliced)
2 hard-boiled eggs (sliced)
1 packet leek soup
1 pint water

Break the cauliflower into pieces. Arrange with the carrots and eggs in layers in a casserole. Make up the leek soup as directed on the packet using the pint of water. Pour over the ingredients in the casserole. Cook in a hot oven 400°F/Gas 6 for 20 minutes.

Serves 4

19

SAVOURY LUNCHEON MEAT

6 ounces pork luncheon meat
Packet cheese sauce
¼ pint milk
1 ounce Cheddar cheese (grated)
1 ounce breadcrumbs

Cut the luncheon meat into slices or cubes and arrange in a shallow dish. Make up half the packet of cheese sauce with the milk and pour over the luncheon meat. Mix the breadcrumbs and cheese together and sprinkle over the top. Cook in a moderate oven 375°F/Gas 5 for about 20 minutes or until the top is crisp and coloured.

Serves 2

41

BAKED CHICKEN AND PEACH

1 large (1-pound) packet frozen beans
½ pound cooked chicken (cut into pieces)
4 ounces Cheddar cheese (grated)
1 packet savoury white sauce
½ pint milk
3 tablespoons single cream (or top of milk)
1 can sliced peaches

Arrange the beans, chicken, and 3 ounces of the cheese in layers in an oven dish. Make up the white sauce as directed on the packet, stir in the cream and pour over the ingredients in the dish. Bake in a moderate oven 325°F/Gas 3 for 20 minutes. Remove from the oven. Drain peaches well and arrange them over the top of the dish, sprinkle with the rest of the cheese and return to the oven for a further 15 minutes.

Serves 4

69

Entertaining

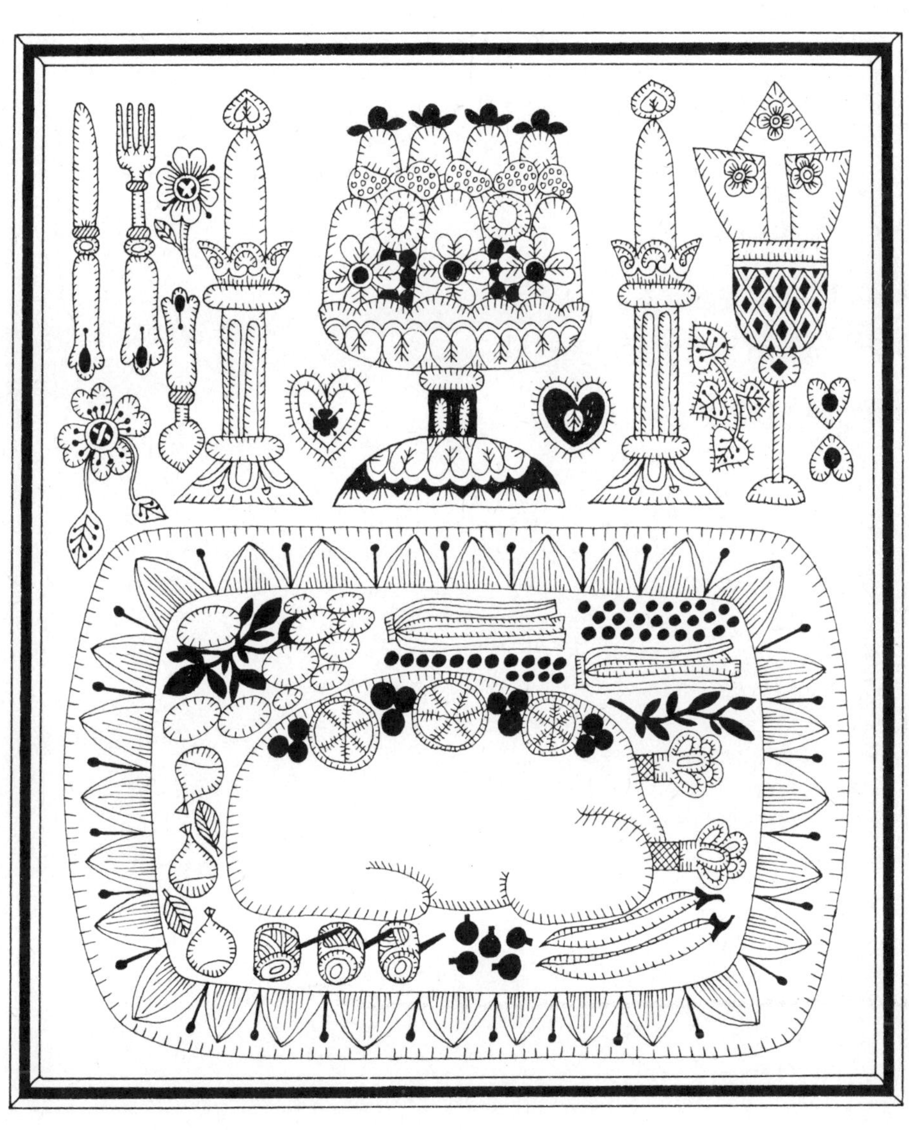

Even if your guests are all, like you, watching their weight they will enjoy these delicious dishes, many from overseas. All the ingredients are easy to obtain.

DUCK WITH BANANAS

1 duck cut into serving pieces
4 tablespoons corn oil (for basting)
Small (8-ounce) tin pineapple slices
1 glass dry red wine
Seasoning
4 bananas
Lemon juice
Sweet potatoes (optional)*

*1 point per ounce extra

Sauce:
Juices from duck, made up to ½ pint with water
Juice and grated rind 1 orange
Chopped pineapple slices
½ ounce cornflour

Place the duck in a roasting pan and brush well with corn oil. Pour the juice from the pineapple into the pan with red wine, salt and pepper, and cook in a moderate oven 375°F/Gas 5 for 40 minutes, or until well cooked, basting frequently with the juices. Place the bananas, unpeeled, in an ovenproof dish, brush with corn oil, sprinkle with lemon juice and bake in a moderate oven for 10 minutes. Serve duck with bananas, sweet potatoes and the sauce.

Sauce: Mix cornflour to a paste with the orange juice. Skim fat from pan juices, reheat and blend with the cornflour. Return to the pan and cook until thick. Add grated rind of orange and pineapple chunks and cook 3 minutes.

Serves 4

129

APRICOT SHOULDER

1 shoulder (about 2 pounds) New Zealand lamb
1 ounce fat or dripping
2 small onions (sliced)
¼ pound dried apricots
2 medium potatoes (peeled and diced)
½ teaspoon rosemary
1 tablespoon flour
¾ pint stock or water
Salt and pepper

Cut the meat into cubes, removing any excess fat and skin. Lightly fry in the fat with the prepared and sliced onions. Remove to a casserole and mix the meat with the dried apricots and half the peeled and diced potato and rosemary. Stir the flour into the fat in the pan and cook for a few minutes. Stir in the stock and seasoning, then pour into the casserole. Sprinkle the remaining diced potato on top. Cover and cook in a moderate oven, 350°F/Gas 4, for about 1 hour. Remove the lid, raise the temperature to 400°F/Gas 6, and continue cooking until the potatoes are browned.

Serves 4

92

OLD ENGLISH PIE

¾ pound stewing steak
¼ pound ox kidney
1 ounce seasoned flour
2 tablespoons oil
2 ounces mushrooms
1 small onion
1 small clove garlic
Pinch dry mustard
1 small teaspoon brown table sauce
1 bouquet garni
1 small hard-boiled egg
Salt
Black pepper (finely ground)

Pastry:
6 ounces plain flour
2½ ounces lard
1½ ounces margarine
Some beaten egg
Little cold water

Trim the meat, remove the core from the kidney and cut into 1-inch squares; roll in flour, shaking in a sieve to remove the surplus. Sauté the meat in the oil until browned on all sides. Drain. Rough chop the mushrooms, finely chop onion and garlic, mingle these with the meat and put in a heavy saucepan with a well-fitting lid, add seasoning, table sauce and bouquet garni and scarcely cover with meat stock or water with a bouillon cube added. Bring to the boil, then cook very slowly for 1½–2 hours until the meat is tender. Thicken with a mixture of cornflour and water if required. Pour into pie dish, distribute sliced hard-boiled egg over the top and cool. Cover with a rich shortcrust pastry, baked at 400°F/Gas 6 for 20–25 minutes. The quality of the pastry is much improved if given an hour in the refrigerator prior to rolling out.

Serves 4

127

LIVER AND BACON LOAF

8 ounces lambs' liver (finely chopped)
4 ounces streaky bacon (derinded and finely chopped, reserving two rashers)
1 medium onion (peeled and finely chopped)
1 egg (beaten)
1 tablespoon brown sauce
Salt
Pepper
1 packet onion and mushroom stuffing
1 ounce butter

Prepare the stuffing as instructed on the packet beating in the egg and the brown sauce. Season well. Lightly fry the onion, bacon and liver in melted butter, remove from pan and combine with stuffing. Grease a 1-pound loaf tin and line the base with the two rashers of streaky bacon. Transfer the mixture to the tin, smooth the top and bake for one hour at 375°F/Gas 5.
This can be served hot for one meal and cold with salad at another meal.

Serves 4

48½

OLD FASHIONED PORK AND APPLE MOULD

Stock:
1 pork bone (trimmed of excess fat)
1 onion (sliced)
$1\frac{1}{2}$ pints water
1 tablespoon herbs

1 pound lean pork fillet
$\frac{1}{4}$ level teaspoon ground ginger
$\frac{3}{4}$ level teaspoon ground cinnamon
1 level teaspoon paprika pepper
Salt and pepper to taste
2 tablespoons oil
$\frac{1}{2}$ ounce gelatine dissolved in 2 tablespoons water
1 large cooking apple (peeled, cored and diced)
1 tablespoon peas (cooked)

Garnish:
Onion rings
Tomato slices
Watercress

Place pork bone, onions and herbs in water in a saucepan. Bring to boil. Cover and simmer gently for 30 minutes. Cut meat into small pieces and mix with spices and seasonings. Strain stock and return to pan. Sauté the pork in the fat until browned on all sides. Drain and stir the meat pieces into the stock and cook for 40–45 minutes, or until tender. Add the dissolved gelatine. When nearly set add diced apple and peas and pour mixture into a basin or mould. Refrigerate for several hours, or until set. To serve, unmould and garnish with watercress, onion rings and tomato slices.

Serves 6

69

PIQUANT VEAL ESCALOPES

2 escalopes, about 4 ounces each, of veal (well pounded)
1 ounce flour
1 ounce butter
2 thin rashers bacon
2 ounces Gruyère cheese
2 tablespoons single cream
1 teaspoon mild mustard

Flatten the veal well by banging with the end of a wooden rolling pin. Dip escalopes in flour. Heat the butter and fry the escalopes until brown on both sides; put them in a shallow oven dish. On each one put a slice of bacon and on the bacon put slice of cheese, pressing lightly together. Bake in a fairly hot oven, 400°F/Gas 6 for about 20 minutes, by which time the bacon should be cooked and the cheese melted. Blend the cream with the mustard and pour over the meat, cook for 5 minutes longer.

Serves 2

46

CHINESE SWEET AND SOUR LAMB CUTLETS

2 lamb cutlets (or 4 baby lamb chops)
Seasoning
1 pear (peeled, cored and sliced)
1 dessertspoon lemon juice
Peas to garnish (2 tablespoons)

Sweet and sour sauce:
½ the juice from one tin pineapple chunks
1 carrot (chopped and cooked)
½ green pepper (sliced and cooked)
½ level tablespoon cornflour
½ tablespoon brown sugar
2 teaspoons soy sauce
1 tablespoon olive oil
1½ tablespoons vinegar
2 gherkins (sliced)
Coarsely grated rind half orange

Sprinkle the meat with seasoning and grill the cutlets or chops, 4 minutes on each side. Keep warm. Marinate pear slices in lemon juice. Heat the pineapple juice with green pepper and carrot. Blend cornflour and sugar with a little cold water, add to the hot fruit juice, return to heat and thicken. Add soy sauce, olive oil, vinegar, gherkins and orange rind and reheat. Arrange cutlets in centre of dish, garnish with cutlet frills. Place pears and peas around cutlets. Mask cutlets and pears with sweet and sour sauce.

Serves 2

54

DANISH GRYDERET (STEW) WITH RAVIOLI

2 tablespoons olive oil
1½ ounces butter
1 medium onion (chopped)
Pinch of sugar
1 medium green pepper (sliced)
3 medium tomatoes (skinned and quartered)
2 ounces button mushrooms (fresh or canned)
2 ounces streaky bacon (cut into 1-inch squares)
1 8-ounce can Danish party sausages (drained)
¾ pound pork fillet (trimmed and cut into 1-inch cubes)
Salt, pepper and paprika to taste
⅓ tablespoon caraway seeds (optional)
1 15¼-ounce can Danish ravioli

Preheat the oil and butter in a frying pan. Add the onion. Cook this until it begins to turn golden brown—adding a pinch of sugar to make them crisp. Add the peppers, tomatoes and mushrooms and cook for a further 4–5 minutes. Stir the mixture from time to time so that the onion does not become over-cooked. Transfer ingredients from pan to a fireproof dish and keep hot.

Fry the bacon (in the same frying pan) and when it is beginning to turn crisp add about three-quarters of the Danish party sausages. Cook for a few minutes, with the bacon, until sausages are lightly browned. Remove ingredients from pan and put with vegetables in dish to keep hot.

Quickly fry cubes of pork for 4–6 minutes, adding more oil or butter if necessary. Season with salt, pepper and paprika. Return vegetables, bacon and sausages to pork in pan. Scatter caraway seeds over, and continue cooking for a further 5–8 minutes, until well heated through. Serve at once with the ravioli—previously heated according to directions given on the can—as accompaniment.

Serves 4

106

TASTY ROLL UP

1 lean loin of pork (boned and rolled)
2 ounces butter
Juice ½ lemon
Seasoning
1 large tin whole figs (12 in syrup)
3 pears (peeled, cored and quartered)
Lemon rind (coarsely grated)

Place pork in roasting tin. Dot the surface with butter, sprinkle with lemon juice and season. Roast in a hot oven, 425°F/Gas 7, for 20–25 minutes, then reduce heat to 375°F/Gas 5 for further 40 minutes. Place pork in a shallow casserole and add the figs and pears. Return to the oven for a further half hour. Serve sprinkled with coarsely grated lemon rind.

Serves 6

201

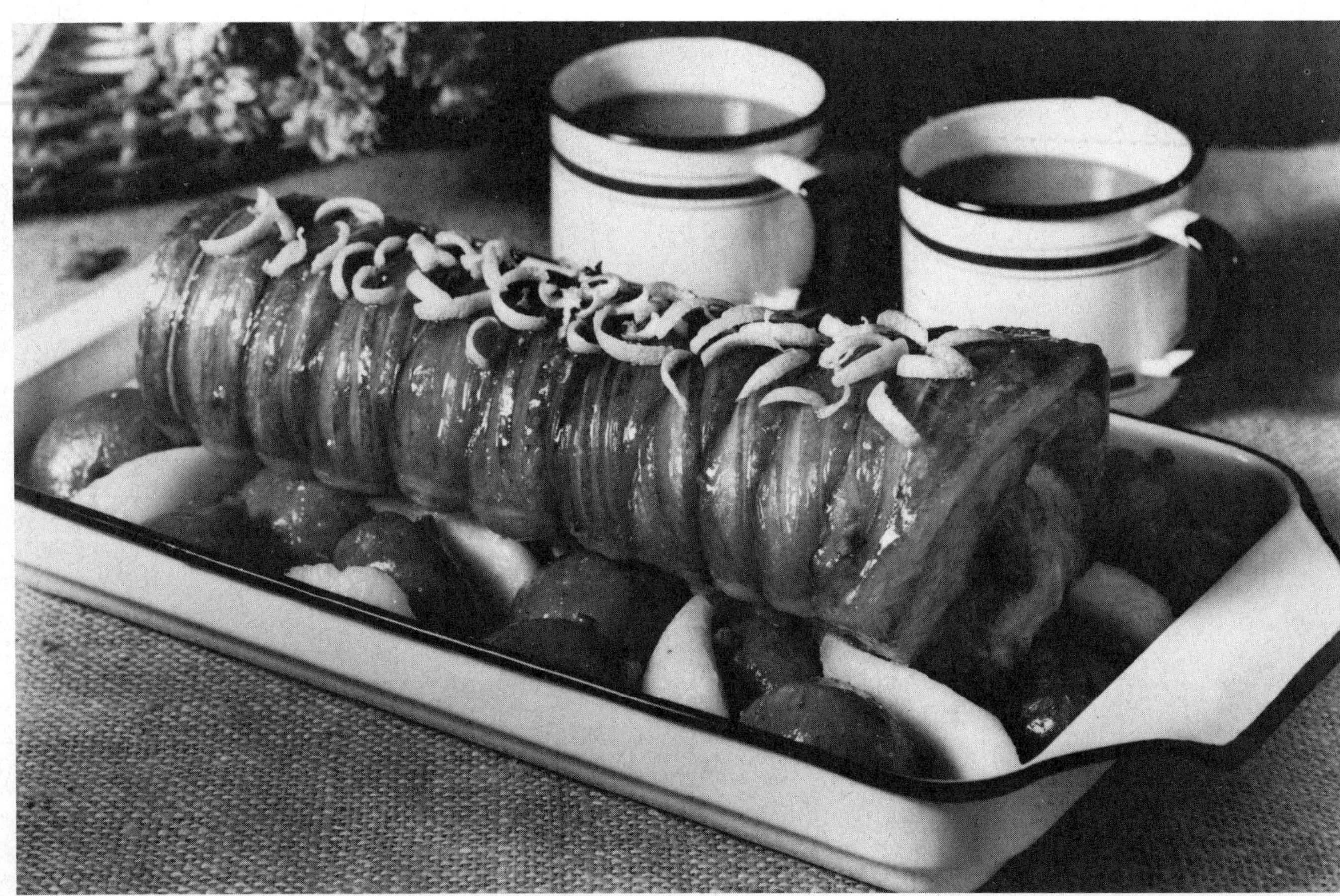

CZECHOSLOVAKIAN STEW WITH BREADCRUMB DUMPLINGS

$\frac{1}{4}$ pound carrots
2 sticks celery
2–3 tablespoons of oil
$\frac{1}{2}$ ounce butter
1 large onion (quartered) or 6 button onions
$\frac{3}{4}$ pound stewing veal
1 ounce seasoned flour
$\frac{1}{2}$ pint stock made with a chicken stock cube
Pinch of mace
$\frac{1}{2}$ tablespoon parsley (finely chopped)
Little rind and juice from a lemon

Dumplings:
4 ounces fresh white breadcrumbs
2 tablespoons milk
1 ounce butter or margarine
Little beaten egg
About $\frac{1}{2}$ teaspoon salt, pepper

Cut carrots and celery into $\frac{1}{4}$-inch slices. Heat oil and butter in a medium-sized saucepan. Add vegetables, cover with a lid and cook gently, without browning for 10 minutes. Cut veal into $\frac{1}{2}$-inch cubes, toss in seasoned flour. Add to vegetables and cook quickly until sealed, stirring frequently. Add stock, mace and parsley and bring to the boil. Turn down and simmer for approximately 40 minutes or turn into an ovenproof dish and bake in a moderate oven, 350°F/ Gas 4, for about 40 minutes. Add lemon juice and rind just before serving.

Dumplings: Soak breadcrumbs in milk. Warm butter then beat in egg and soaked breadcrumbs, add salt and pepper. Shape into 4 small balls. Cook dumplings in boiling salted water for 5 minutes. Drain and add to stew about 10 minutes before the end of its cooking time.

Serves 2

74½

SOUTH PACIFIC PORK AND PINEAPPLE

$\frac{1}{2}$ pound lean pork fillet
1 dessertspoon seasoned flour
1 tart eating apple (cored and diced)
3 tablespoons oil
$\frac{1}{2}$ clove garlic (crushed)
1 small tin pineapple pieces
Small leek (sliced and blanched)
Small green pepper (thinly sliced and seeds removed)
Salt and pepper to taste

Cut pork into 1-inch cubes, mix with flour and seasoning. Heat oil with garlic; fry pork until lightly browned on all sides. Lower heat and add apples, pineapple pieces, leek and green pepper. Adjust seasoning. Continue cooking over gentle heat for 15–20 minutes, or until tender.

Serves 2

53

SCANDINAVIAN BURGERS

6 ounces lean minced steak
4 ounces lean ham (finely diced)
2 ounces onion (finely chopped)
$\frac{1}{2}$ teaspoon salt
$\frac{1}{8}$ teaspoon pepper
1 ounce blue cheese
$\frac{1}{4}$ pint dry red wine
1 tablespoon pure vegetable oil for shallow frying
1 tablespoon flour

Mix the minced steak, ham, onions, salt and pepper. Divide the mince mixture and the cheese into two parts. Form into round cakes, placing the cheese in the centre. Pour the wine over the burgers and allow to stand for at least three hours, turning the burgers over from time to time. Heat the oil and lightly brown the burgers all over, reduce the heat, cover and fry for 7 minutes on both sides. Remove the burgers to a serving dish and keep hot. Stir the flour into the pure vegetable oil and then add the wine, stirring well, cook for 1 minute. Pour the stock over the burgers and serve.

Serves 2

45

MEXICAN CHILI CON CARNE

1 dessertspoon pure vegetable oil for shallow frying
$\frac{1}{2}$ pound minced beef
$\frac{1}{2}$ pound onions (chopped)
1 clove garlic (crushed)
6 ounces tomatoes (skinned and chopped)
About $\frac{1}{4}$ ounce chili powder to taste
1 small green pepper (sliced)
2 ounces red kidney beans (soaked overnight)
Pinch salt
$\frac{1}{4}$ pint water or stock
$\frac{1}{2}$ ounce flour
2 tablespoons stock

Heat the pure vegetable oil and sauté the minced beef, onion and garlic until browned. Add the tomatoes, chili powder, green pepper, red kidney beans, salt and stock. Cover and simmer gently for 35 minutes, stirring occasionally to prevent sticking. Mix the flour with the remaining stock and blend into the mixture, then cook for a further 5 minutes.

Serves 2

41

NORWEGIAN RAW SPICED HERRINGS

2 salted herrings
$\frac{1}{4}$ pint tarragon vinegar
2 tablespoons sugar
$\frac{1}{4}$ pint tomato juice
4 cloves
4 allspice
1 gherkin (chopped)
1 small onion (chopped)
2 bay leaves

Soak herrings in cold water overnight. Mix the other ingredients to make a marinade and leave to stand for a few hours. Clean and fillet herrings, cut in $\frac{1}{2}$-inch slices. Pour marinade over them. Serve next day, chilled.

Serves 2

27$\frac{1}{2}$

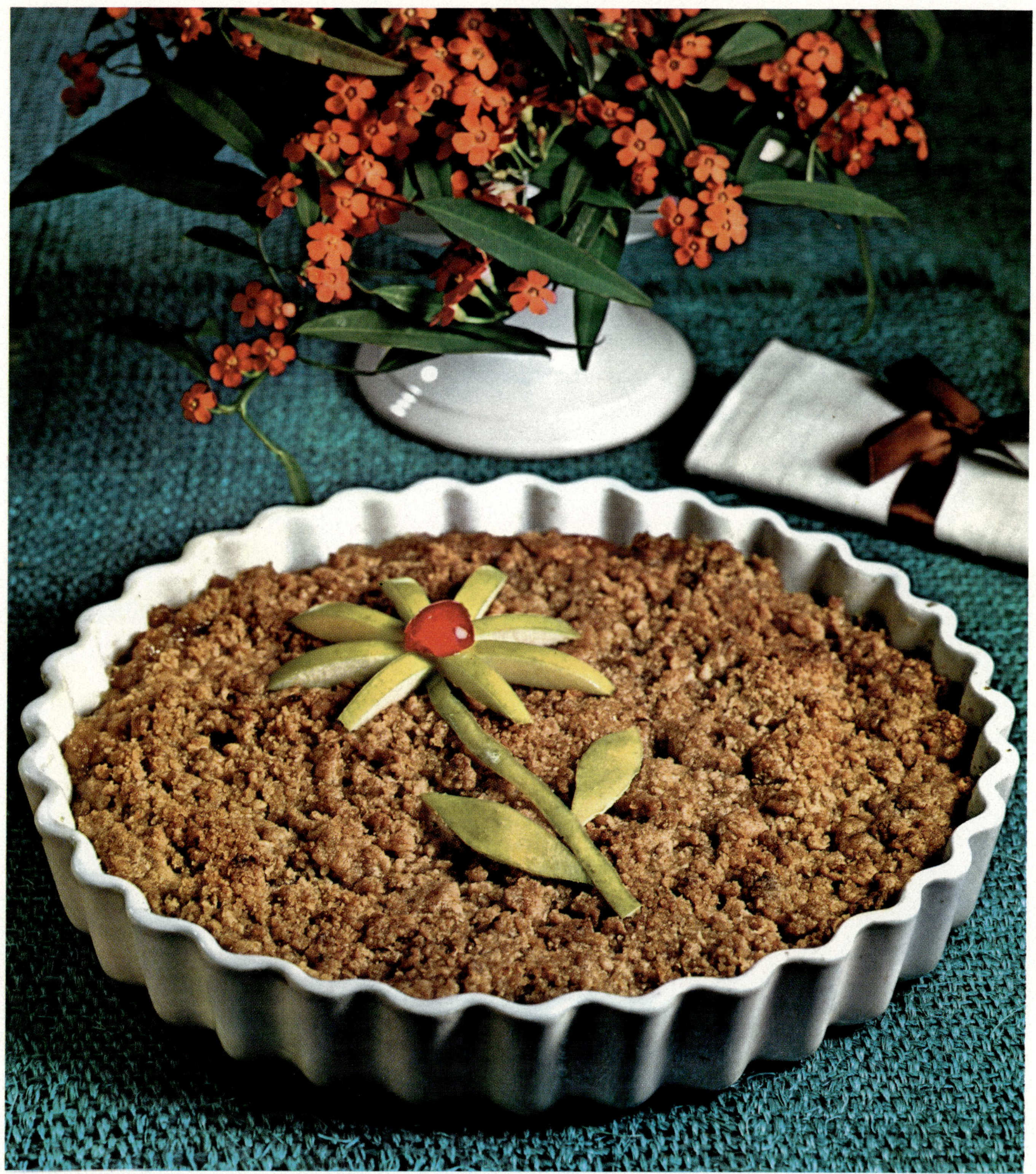

Apple Crisp – a decorative addition to any table (page 66)

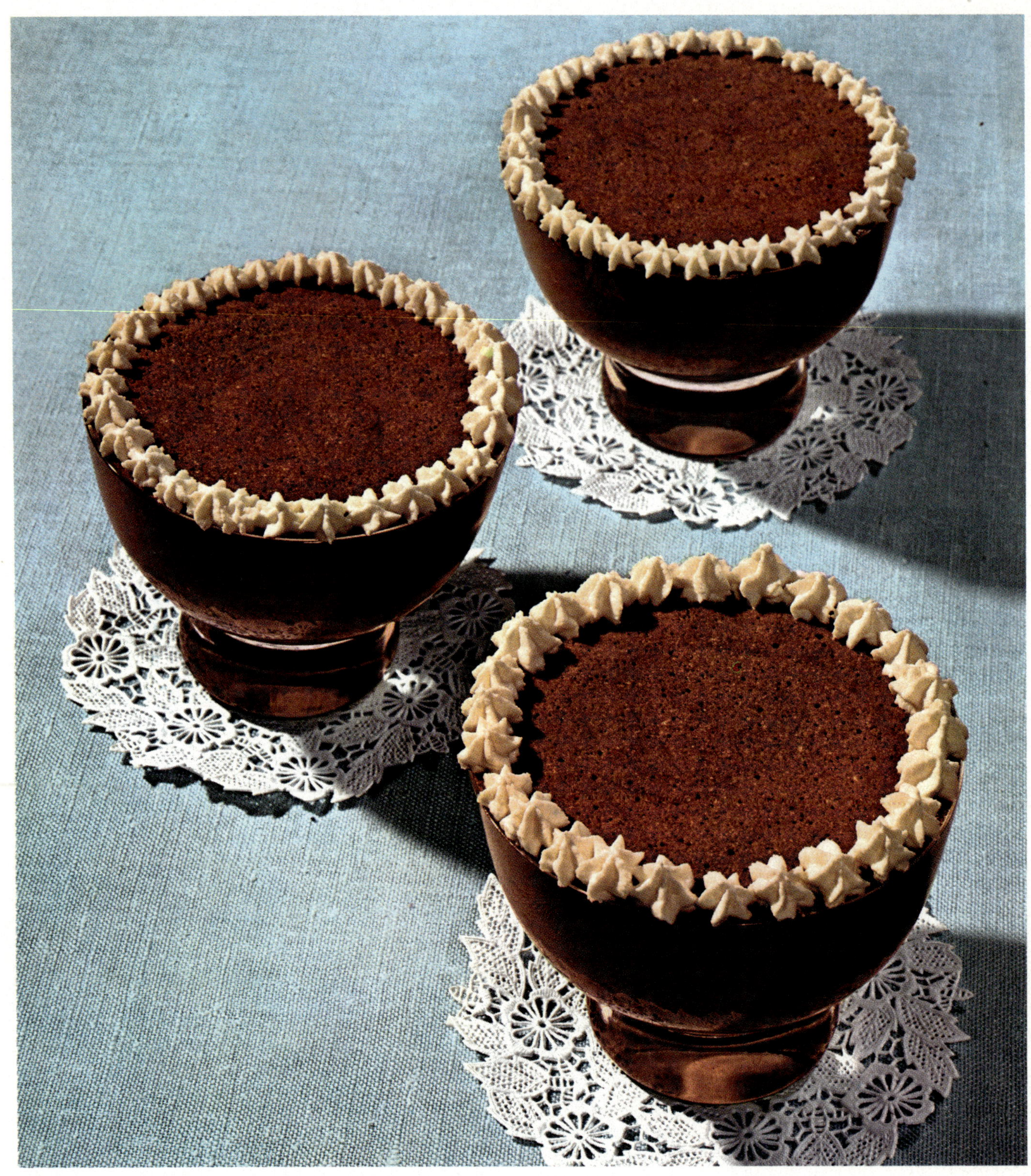

Chocolate Mousse – a lower points-rating than you might think (see page 67)

TURKISH FOUDJA DJEDAD 007

(One of James Bond's favourite recipes)

2 large cooking apples
2 ounces cooked chicken
Salt and pepper
1 ounce breadcrumbs
1 ounce dried raisins
2 ounces mushrooms
½ ounce chopped nuts
6 cloves
Pinch saffron
Pinch cinnamon
Pinch ginger
½ tablespoon butter

Remove the core of the apples. Chop up the chicken and mix with the mushrooms, salt, pepper and breadcrumbs. Mix the melted butter with the cloves, raisins, ginger, cinnamon and chopped nuts. Add to the chicken mixture and fill the apples with the mixture. Put a little brown sugar and a dab of butter on each apple. Score round the centre of each apple to prevent them from bursting.
Cover the bottom of a baking dish with boiling water. Place the apples in the dish and bake in a medium oven, 350°F/Gas 4, for half an hour.

Serves 2

29

CORSICAN TRUITES AUX AMANDES

2 trout
Little oil
1 ounce butter
2 tablespoons lemon juice
¼ level teaspoon black pepper
2 ounce almonds (blanched and toasted)
Parsley

If frozen trout, thaw thoroughly. Place the trout on the greased rack of the grillpan and brush with oil. Grill gently for 10–15 minutes in all, turning once half way through the cooking time. Remove from the grill and put on a serving dish to keep warm. Add the lemon juice, black pepper and almonds to the melted butter in the grill pan and heat through. Pour over the trout and serve.

Serves 2

32

FRENCH VICHYSSOISE

3 large leeks
2 ounces butter
2 medium-size potatoes
¾ pint chicken stock made with stock cube
Salt and pepper
Little grated nutmeg
¼ pint double cream
Some chives (finely chopped)

Cut the green part from the leeks, then cut the white parts into 1-inch lengths. Sauté these white parts in butter until soft, but do not let them brown. Peel and slice the potatoes and add to the leeks with the stock. Season to taste and add nutmeg. Simmer until the vegetables are soft. Sieve the vegetables and stock through a fine sieve (or blend in an electric blender). Chill well. Add the cream just before serving, and serve sprinkled with chopped chives.

Serves 4

59

SPANISH VEAL CUTLETS

2 large veal cutlets
2 slices Cheddar cheese
Beaten egg
Breadcrumbs
Fat for frying

With a very sharp knife slice the veal cutlets open, leaving one end uncut. Open the cutlet and place a piece of cheese inside. Dip the cutlets in beaten egg and breadcrumbs and deep fry till golden brown. Serve with vegetables (*see* page 103 for points).

Serves 2

34

FRENCH PIPERADE

6 ounces onion (chopped)
1½ ounces butter
½ dessertspoon olive oil
1 large green pepper (cut into strips)
½ pound tomatoes (skinned and chopped)
Large pinch basil
Seasoning
3 eggs
2 tablespoons fresh double cream
2 lean gammon rashers (about 4 ounces each)

Fry the onions gently in the butter and oil until soft but not brown. Add peppers and cook slowly until soft. Add the chopped tomatoes and basil, and season to taste. Cover pan and cook very slowly for 20 minutes. Beat the eggs lightly with the cream and pour over the vegetable mixture. Continue to cook slowly until the eggs are lightly scrambled. Put in a warm serving dish and top with the grilled gammon rashers.

Serves 2

65

Drinks

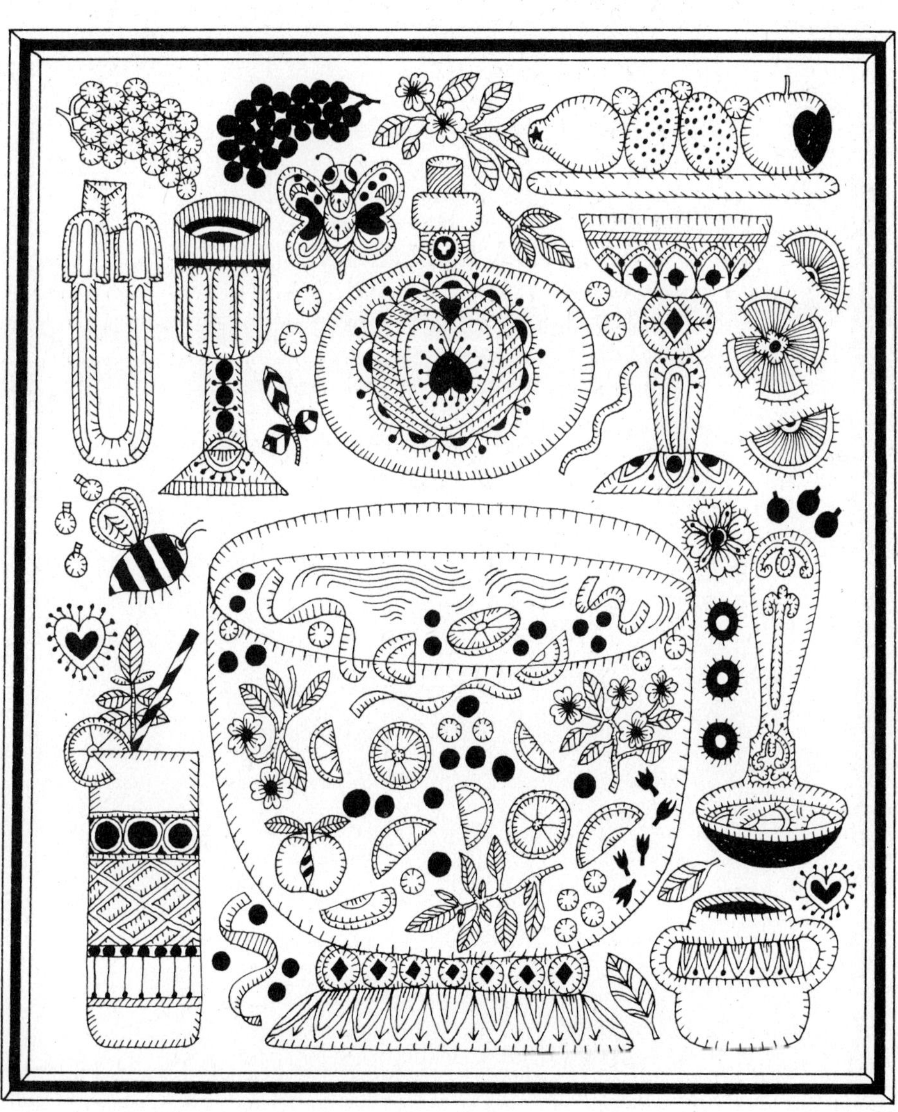

Drinks

It's not strictly true to say that drinks are 'cookery', although I've seen some involved cocktails that took as long to mix as a recipe!

So I make no apology for including this section on drinks. After all, we probably invite friends in 'for a drink' more often than 'for a meal'.

PEP COCKTAIL

Per glass:

1 egg
1 tablespoon clear honey
Juice 1 orange and ½ lemon

Beat egg yolk, honey and fruit juice with beater until fluffy. Fold in egg white, stiffly beaten. Serve.

8½

HOT HONEYED ORANGE

6 oranges
3 lemons
¼–½ pint water
9 level tablespoons clear honey
Cloves

Squeeze the juice from the oranges and lemons, keeping one orange back. Add water and sweeten with the honey. Heat until almost boiling. Pour into mugs. Slice the remaining orange and press few cloves into the centre of each slice. Float an orange slice on top of each mug. In summertime, Honeyed Orange makes a refreshing drink served cold in tall glasses, diluted with an equal volume of chilled soda water.

40½

GOLDEN HARVEST CIDER

1 screwtop flagon Woodpecker Cider
1 pint dry ginger ale
2 oranges
2 lemons
1 miniature bottle orange Curaçao (optional)

Chill the cider and ginger ale. Cut the peel from the oranges and lemons in fairly long strips and put into a large jug with the juice from the fruit. Add the orange Curaçao and leave to stand for 5 minutes. Add the cider and ginger ale.

32

LEMROSE SODA

Per glass:
1 tablespoon rose hip syrup
1 tablespoon lemon barley
Soda water
1 tablespoon ice cream

Stir together in a glass the rose hip syrup and lemon barley, then top up with soda water. Add the ice cream.

5

BANANA ROSE SHAKE

Per glass:
1 brickette ice cream
1 medium ripe banana
1 tablespoon rose hip syrup
$\frac{1}{4}$ pint chilled milk
Few drops vanilla essence

Soften ice cream, mash banana well and mix together. Whisk in rose hip syrup, milk and vanilla essence.

11

ROSANNA CRUSH

Per glass:
1 medium ripe banana
3 dessertspoons rose hip syrup
$\frac{1}{4}$ pint milk
Little ground cinnamon

Mash the banana finely and beat in rose hip syrup. Gradually whisk in the milk and pour into a glass. Dust lightly with cinnamon.

9

GINGER ROSE FIZZ

2 dessertspoons rose hip syrup
½ small bottle ginger beer
1 tablespoon vanilla ice cream

Put the rose hip syrup into a tall glass and top up with ginger beer, stirring lightly. Then float the ice cream on top.

6

HONEY ROSE

Per glass:
1 tablespoon lime cordial
Hot water to mix
1 level teaspoon clear honey
1 dessertspoon rose hip syrup

Pour lime cordial into a beaker, two-thirds full with hot water, then stir in honey and rose hip syrup.

2½

SUNSET NOG

Per glass:
1 large egg
1 ounce caster sugar
1 tablespoon rose hip syrup
Large pinch nutmeg

Put egg, sugar and rose hip syrup into a basin standing over a pan of gently boiling water. Beat continuously until mixture is thick, light in colour and foamy. Pour into a glass. Sprinkle with nutmeg and serve at once.

10

WHITE WINE CUP

1 bottle dry white wine
1 bottle soda water
1 wineglass medium sherry
Rind 1 lemon
1 ounce powdered sugar
Thin slices of fresh pineapple
Mint
$\frac{1}{8}$ bottle brandy ($3\frac{1}{2}$ fluid ounces)
Ice

Mix all ingredients together, garnish with slivers of lemon rind and thin slices of pineapple.

38

GLÜHWEIN

1 bottle dry wine (white or red)
3 small sticks cinnamon
6 cloves
$\frac{1}{4}$ pound sugar
6 slices orange peel
6 slices lemon peel

Mix all ingredients in a pot. Heat gently on a very low heat and bring to near boiling point.

38

HOT WINE PUNCH

1 bottle dry wine (red or white)
$\frac{1}{2}$ pint water
3 teaspoons sugar
6 cloves
3 small pieces stick cinnamon
Rind of 1 lemon (cut very fine)

Boil the three teaspoons of sugar in the water, add the cloves, cinnamon and lemon rind. When this comes to the boil, remove from heat and add wine. Serve piping hot.

$23\frac{1}{2}$

FOAMY FRUIT JUICE COCKTAIL

¼ pint water
2 ounces granulated sugar
¼ pint lemon juice (fresh or unsweetened bottled)
¼ pint orange juice (fresh or unsweetened bottled)
¼ pint lime juice (bottled)
2 eggs
2 cups ice (finely crushed)

Put water and sugar in a small pan and heat till the sugar has dissolved. Allow to cool. Put all ingredients into a shaker (or jar with a screw top) and shake until frothy. Pour into glasses and serve.

21

Silhouette Recipes

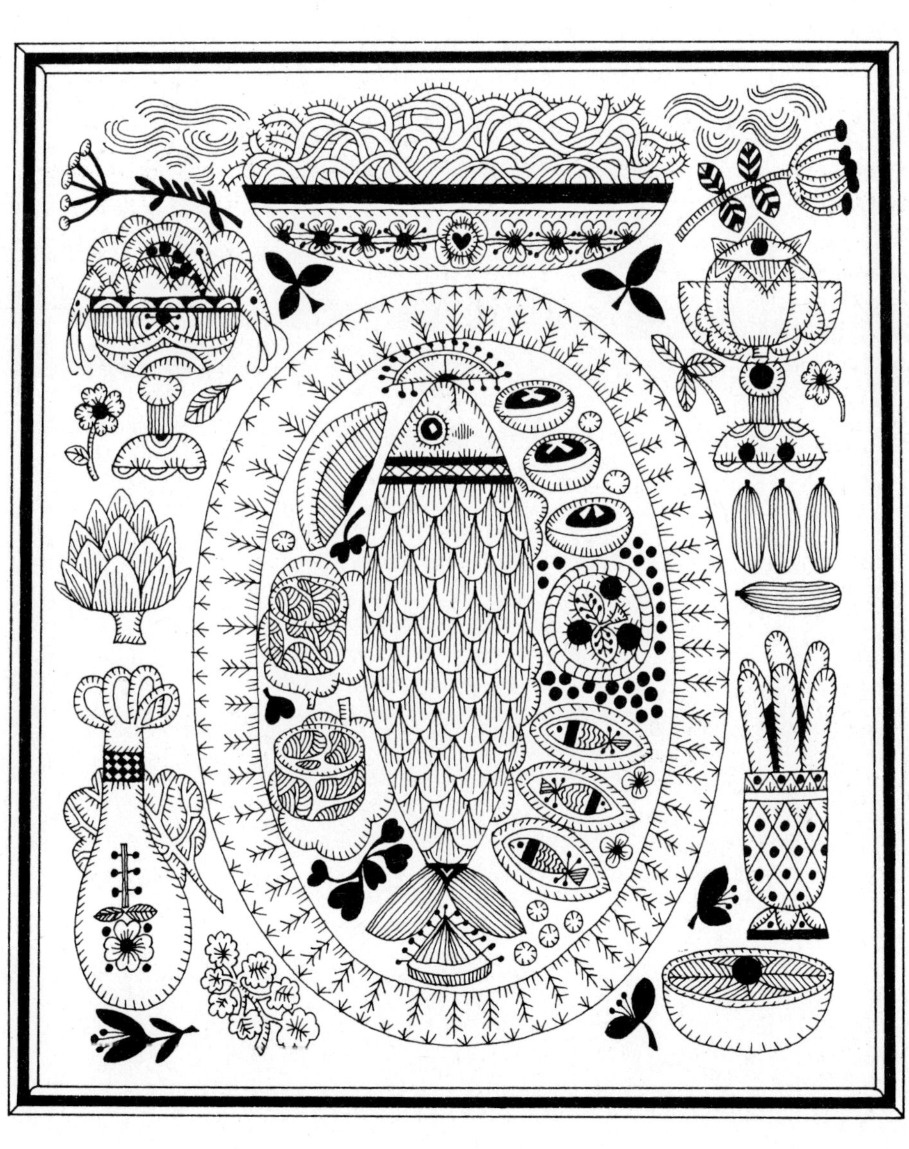

Silhouette Recipes

Here we reproduce a selection of recipes sent in by Silhouette members, who have found them extremely useful in their own battles against weight.

SLIMMERS' SOUP

½ pound onions
½ pound tomatoes (skinned)
½ pound carrots
6 stalks celery
½ ounce butter
Salt and pepper
2½ pints stock made from stock cubes

Peel and dice all the vegetables. Sauté onions in butter until lightly brown. Add diced vegetables, stock and salt and pepper to taste. Bring to boil then simmer for 20 minutes or until vegetables are tender.

Serves 4

Anne Dickens, Northampton Class

5

GRAPEFRUIT AND ORANGE COCKTAIL

1 orange
1 grapefruit

Cut the orange and grapefruit in half across and scoop out the pulp of each with a teaspoon. Mix and pile back into the grapefruit halves. Chill and serve.

Serves 2

Mrs. H. Milne, Fraserburgh Class

3

MAXIMILIENNE EGGS

2 large tomatoes
2 eggs
1 ounce grated Cheddar cheese

Cut the tops of the tomatoes and scoop out the centres. Drop an egg into each tomato shell and top with grated cheese. Place on a baking tray and cook in a medium oven for about 5 minutes, or until eggs are set and cheese melted.

Serves 2

Mrs. Adams, Edinburgh Class

13

CHEESE STUFFED EGG

Per person:
1 hard-boiled egg
1 ounce grated cheese
Pinch pepper
Pinch salt
1 tablespoon milk

Cut the hard-boiled egg in half lengthwise. Scoop out the yolk and mash with a fork. Mix the cheese, seasoning and milk with the masked yolk and pile the mixture into the whites. Serve on crisp lettuce.

Mrs. A. Harvey, Rugeley Class

8

FILLET OF SOLE WITH MUSHROOM SAUCE

3–4 ounces fillets sole
¾ teaspoon salt
Little white pepper
½ tablespoon butter or margarine
¼ pound mushrooms (thinly sliced)
½ onion (chopped)
¼ cup dry white wine
1 teaspoon flour
3 dessertspoons single cream
1 tablespoon chopped parsley

Sprinkle the fillets with salt and pepper. Melt the butter and sauté half the sliced mushroom and onion for three minutes. Lay the seasoned fillets on top of this mixture and cover with remaining mushrooms. Pour the wine over them, cover and simmer over a medium heat for 15 minutes, or until the fish is white and flaky. Mix flour into cream until smooth and add to fish, stirring until thickened. Cook for 2–3 minutes. Serve sprinkled with parsley.

Serves 3

Mrs. M. Astbury, Rugeley Class

6

CHICKEN WITH ORANGE

2 joints chicken
1 large orange
1 dessertspoon Worcestershire sauce
Salt and pepper

Pre-heat oven to 375°F/Gas 5. Wash chicken joints and place in an ovenproof casserole. Season lightly with salt and pepper. Squeeze juice from orange and pour the juice over the chicken, together with Worcestershire sauce. Cover and cook for 1½–2 hours (until chicken is tender), basting only once with juice. To serve, place on dish and pour over all the sauce remaining in the casserole. This should be served with green vegetables or a green salad.

Serves 2

Mrs. J. Brailsford, Eastwood Class

15

BEEFBURGER BOLOGNAISE

4 ounces spaghetti
2 beefburgers
1 onion (finely sliced)
½ ounce butter
1 4-ounce can peeled tomatoes
Cup water
Salt and pepper
Parmesan cheese (optional)

Cook the spaghetti in boiling salted water for 15 minutes. Meanwhile, grill beefburgers. Cook onions in large pan, add tomatoes, water and seasoning and simmer whilst the spaghetti finishes cooking. Drain the spaghetti, place on serving dish and coat with the sauce. Place beefburgers on top and sprinkle with cheese, if liked.

Serves 2

Mrs. J. Webster and *Mrs. P. Damp, Leyland Class*

38

BEEF AND VEGETABLE MEDLEY

6 ounces minced beef
1 medium carrot
1 stalk celery
1 small onion
2 ounces mushrooms
1 medium size tomato (skinned and sliced)
1 teaspoon salt
1 teaspoon vegetable extract
1 teaspoon Worcestershire sauce
Small cup water

Cook minced beef in stew pan slowly for 10 minutes, add water, sliced carrot, celery, onion, mushrooms and tomato, salt, vegetable extract and Worcestershire sauce. Simmer for 45 minutes. Serve with green beans.

Serves 2

Mrs. Ruth Merchant, Broadstone Class

22

CHEESE SURPRISE

Per person:
1-ounce slice bread (without crusts)
½ ounce narrow Cheddar cheese slices
1 egg
½ rasher bacon (optional)

Set oven to 375°F/Gas 5. Place bread on baking sheet and put cheese slices on the bread around the edges leaving free a square in the centre. Separate the egg yolk and place this in the centre square on the bread. Whisk egg white until firm and spread evenly over the whole slice, sealing edges well. If using bacon, cut it into narrow strips and decorate top of egg with criss-cross strips of bacon.
Place in the centre of the oven and cook until lightly browned—10–12 minutes.

Mrs. M. Styles, Wollaton Class

11

SALMON KEDGEREE

Half 7-ounce can salmon with juice
3 ounces cooked rice
1 egg (hard-boiled)
2 tomatoes
Parsley or chives (chopped)

Place salmon, juice, rice and chopped egg in a basin, season and mix well. Place mixture in a shallow ovenproof dish, top with sliced tomatoes, cover with foil and bake for 20 minutes at 325° F/Gas 3.

Serves 2

Mrs. Joan Jaeger, Southport Class

14

CHEESE AND TOMATO BAKE

3 tomatoes
1 egg
1 ounce Cheddar grated cheese

Cut the tomatoes in half and place the halves in a shallow ovenproof dish (or casserole lid). Cook for 15 minutes at 350°F/Gas 4. Grate the cheese and mix with the lightly beaten egg. Pour egg mixture over tomatoes, pop back into the oven until the egg is set and the top beginning to brown.

Serves 2

Mrs. Edna Stoodley, Taunton Class

5½

CORNED BEEF MASH

Per Person:
2 ounces potato
4 ounces carrot
2 ounces corned beef
1 tomato
6 sprouts
1 6 × 6-inch square foil

Cook potato and sliced carrot together. When cooked strain off water and mash potato and carrot with corned beef. Place mixture on a square of foil. Slice tomato into four and lay slices on top of mixture. Grill under fairly hot grill for 3 or 4 minutes. Serve with sprouts, freshly cooked.

Mrs. Peggy Bannister, Rugeley Class

9½

PRAWN AND PINEAPPLE COLESLAW

$\frac{1}{2}$ small white cabbage
$\frac{1}{2}$ onion
1 red eating apple
Tablespoon lemon juice
1 carrot, grated
$1\frac{1}{2}$ tablespoons mayonnaise
$\frac{1}{2}$ tin sweetcorn
Small tin pineapple cubes
4 ounces prawns
1 tablespoon tomato ketchup
1 tablespoon mayonnaise
Salt and pepper

Finely shred the washed cabbage, add thinly sliced onion and chopped apple (sprinkled with juice of lemon) and the carrot. Place in a bowl and mix well together with drained sweetcorn and mayonnaise.
Drain pineapple cubes and add to prawns. Blend 1 tablespoon of pineapple juice with the tomato ketchup and mayonnaise, and season to taste. Mix with prawns and pineapple. Pile the pineapple mixture in the centre of the coleslaw.

Serves 2

Mrs. P. Sexton, Southampton Class

28

COTTAGE CHEESE SALAD DRESSING

4 ounces cottage cheese
$2\frac{1}{2}$ ounces natural yogurt (unsweetened)
2 gherkins (chopped)
2 stuffed olives (chopped)
Juice 1 orange
Seasonings to taste

Whisk the cottage cheese with the natural yogurt, add the chopped gherkins and olives and stir in the orange juice. Season to taste and chill well before serving.

Serves 2

Mrs. M. Bunting, Leicester Class

$8\frac{1}{2}$

STUFFED CUCUMBER SLICES

1 straight firm cucumber
$\frac{1}{3}$ cup cottage cheese (3 ounces)
1 tablespoon parsley (chopped)
1 tablespoon chili sauce
1 teaspoon Worcestershire sauce

Pare the cucumber and scoop out the centre with a sharp knife. Beat the cottage cheese with the parsley, chili sauce and Worcestershire sauce until well blended and then stuff the mixture into the cavity along the cucumber. Chill and serve cut into $\frac{1}{4}$-inch slices.

Serves 2

Mrs. Astbury Rugeley Class

6

STUFFED COURGETTES

4 small courgettes
1 ounce butter or margarine
½ level teaspoon paprika
2 tomatoes
½ onion (chopped)
¼ pound prawns
Little parmesan cheese
Salt and pepper

Trim off each end of the courgettes. Cook whole for about 5 minutes in boiling salted water. Drain and run cold water over them for a few seconds to preserve the colour. Remove a thin slice lengthways from the courgettes. Carefully scoop out the flesh with a teaspoon, and chop up the flesh. Skin the tomatoes, discard the seeds and chop roughly. Put the butter into a saucepan and add the chopped onion, cook until soft but not brown. Add the paprika, chopped courgette flesh and tomatoes. Season and cook for 3 minutes. Stir in the prawns. Put the courgettes in a buttered gratin dish and fill them with the mixture. Dust with parmesan cheese and brown in a quick oven, 425°F/Gas 7, for 15 minutes.

Serves 4

Mrs. J. Walker, Bradford Class

20½

MARROW IN TOMATO SAUCE

1 medium marrow
½ pound tomatoes (washed and roughly chopped)
1 onion (finely chopped)
1 ounce butter
½ teaspoon rosemary
Pinch thyme
Salt and pepper

Skin, seed and chop marrow.
Sauce: Place all ingredients in a saucepan over a low heat until juices run, when heat can be increased. When tomatoes and onion are quite soft, strain sauce through nylon sieve using a wooden spoon to ensure all liquid is extracted. Return sauce to saucepan and add marrow. Cook until marrow is soft but not mushy.

Serves 2

Mrs. Oliver, Bradford Class

22

EVENING SNACK

¼ pound mushrooms
1 large onion
Salt and pepper to taste
½ eggcup water
½ ounce Cheddar cheese

Wash and slice mushrooms and onion into ovenproof dish. Season with salt and pepper and add water. Cook slowly, 250°F/Gas ½, until onion is cooked. Remove from oven. Grate cheese and spread over the top then pop under a hot grill till cheese is brown and bubbling.

Serves 1

Mrs. Lyn Atherton, Ellesmere Port Class

4½

SILHOUETTE COCKTAIL

2 oranges
1 grapefruit
1 large cooking apple
½ pound grapes
3 egg whites
2 ounces sugar
Glacé cherries to decorate

Peel and cook apple until soft, then put into liquidizer and make into a purée. Leave to cool. Peel the grapefruit and cut into small pieces. Peel the oranges and cut into segments. Wash grapes, remove skin and pips. Mix all the fruit together and place into individual dishes. Whisk egg whites till very stiff. Add the apple purée gently and sweeten mixture with sugar. Pile onto fruit and decorate with glacé cherries.

Serves 4–6

Mrs. L. K. Keane, Denmead Class

27½

FRUIT SALAD IN MELON

1 small melon
1 apple
1 lemon
½ grapefruit
1 peach
1 banana
2 ounces grapes
1 orange
½ pint boiled water (cooled)
2 ounces sugar

Cut melon into two halves crossways, remove seeds. Scoop out as much melon flesh as possible. Leave case. Peel and slice all the fruit, including melon flesh, and place in dish. Squeeze lemon juice over the banana to prevent browning and place the sliced banana with the other fruit. Dissolve sugar in water and add to bowl. Leave to chill in cool place or in refrigerator, when ready to serve pile into melon halves.

Serves 6

Mrs. J. Webster, Leyland Class

25

ORANGE SOUFFLÉ

Grated rind and juice 2 oranges
Juice ½ lemon
½ pint cream for whipping
2 ounces sugar
2 eggs
½ ounce gelatine

Soak gelatine in 4 tablespoons of fruit juice for 5 minutes, warm over hot water until dissolved. Separate eggs, grate rind and squeeze rest of juice from the orange and lemon into a bowl. Whisk egg yolks, sugar, lemon juice and grated rind in a bowl over a pan of hot water until thick and creamy, remove from the heat and continue to whisk. Whip cream lightly and fold into egg mixture; whip the whites and fold these into soufflé; fold in the dissolved gelatine. Pour this mixture into a prepared soufflé dish, chill, decorate with whipped cream.

Serves 4

Mrs. J. Webster, Leyland Class

73½

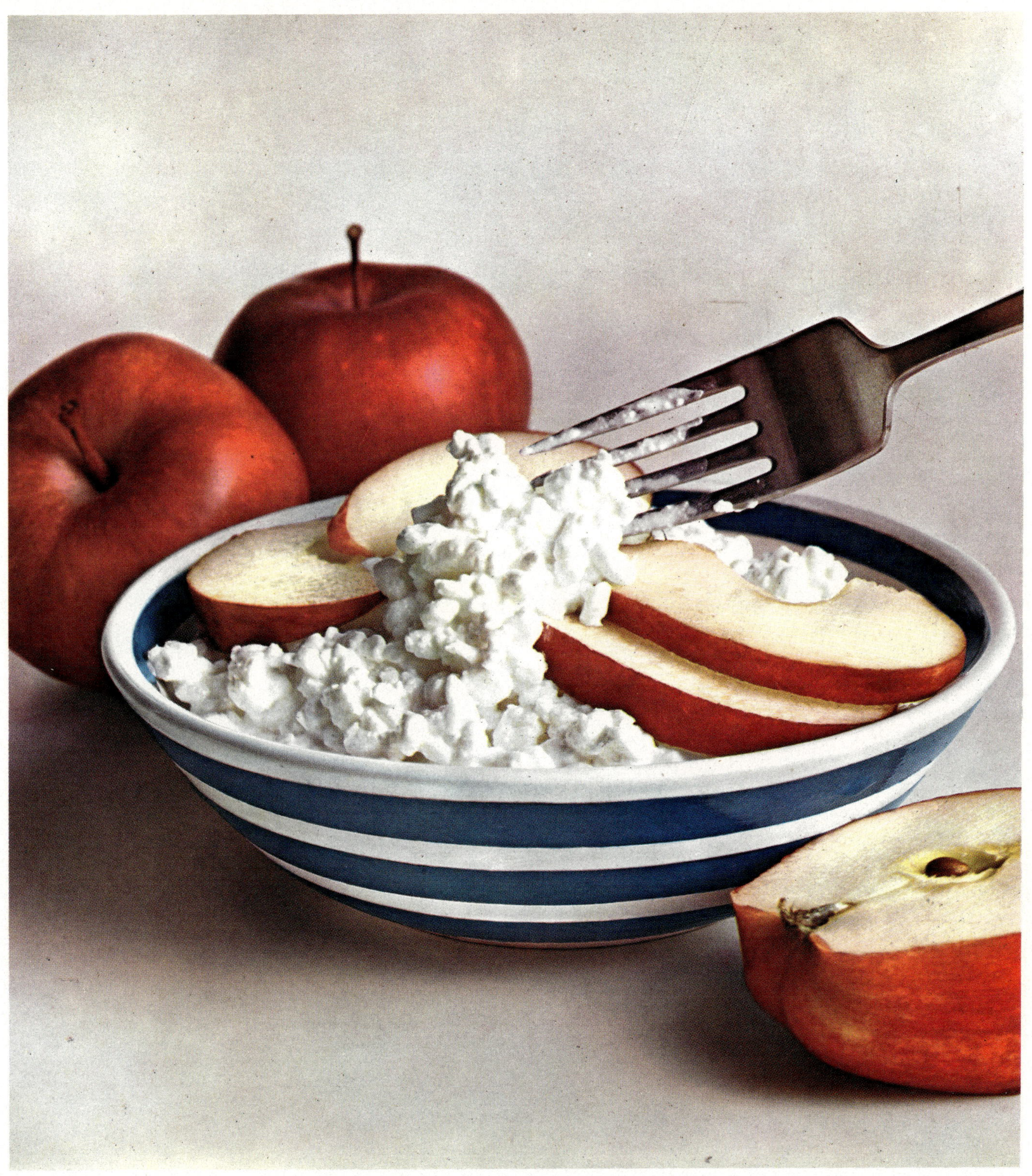

For a really tasty supper snack, try apple slices with cottage cheese

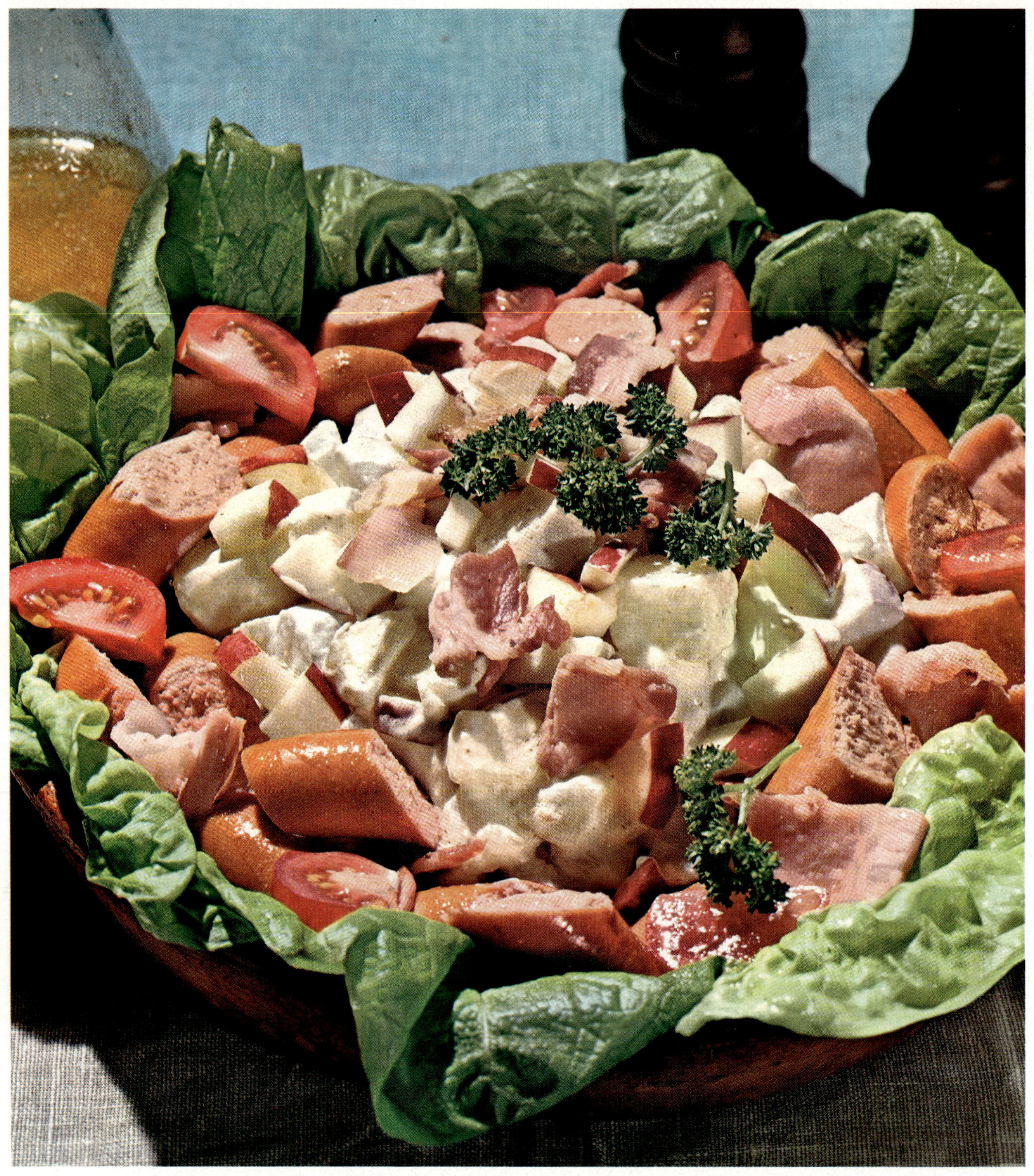

Dress up potato salad with frankfurters, ham and tomatoes for a summer meal the whole family will enjoy

JELLY À LA YOGURT

$\frac{1}{2}$ fruit jelly
$\frac{1}{2}$ pint hot water
1 carton natural yogurt (unsweetened)

Dissolve the jelly in the hot water and allow to cool. When cool pour in the yogurt and stir well.

Serves 2

Mrs. Jean Slatter, Berks, Hants and Dorset Area Manager

10

YOGURT SURPRISE

4 ounces plain low-fat yogurt (unsweetened)
$\frac{1}{2}$ pint apple purée (unsweetened)
4 drops liquid sweetener
Large pinch cinnamon

Blend yogurt with apple purée, cinnamon, and liquid sweetener. Pour into individual glasses and chill before serving.

Serves 2

Mrs. Main, Fraserburgh Class

$10\frac{1}{2}$

PINEAPPLE ICE CREAM

8-ounce carton double cream
Equal quantity of liquidized fresh pineapple
1 tablespoon sugar

Whip cream until thick, add sugar and liquidized fruit (use the cream carton to measure the correct quantity of fruit). Pour mixture in plastic container, cover with lid or foil and place in freezer compartment of refrigerator set at normal temperature. Leave for 2 hours and ice cream is ready to serve.

Serves 10

Mrs. Oliver, Bradford Class

55

RASPBERRY CREAM SLICE

2 crispbreads
¼ ounce butter
1 teaspoon raspberry jam
2 ounces cottage cheese

Spread the crispbreads first with butter and then with jam. Pile the cottage cheese on top. This makes a delightful substitute for a cream cake.

Serves 2

Mrs. Joan Ash, Rugeley Class

8

APPLE SNOW

2 medium-sized cooking apples
2 eggs
1 teaspoon sweetener

Stew apple in a little water and leave to cool. Separate yolk from white of egg. Mix yolk, stewed apple and half the sweetener, and place in a small greased oven dish. Beat egg whites until it forms peaks, stir in the rest of the sweetener and spread over the apple mixture. Bake in a hot oven, 400°F/Gas 6, until topping is golden and crisp.

Serves 2

Mrs. J. F. Cureton, Rugeley Class

12

SLIMMERS SORBET

1–5-ounce carton natural yogurt (unsweetened)
1 orange
1 egg white
½ can Florida orange juice
½ tablespoon gelatine dissolved in 2 tablespoons water
1 fresh orange

Set refrigerator to lowest setting. Combine orange juice and yogurt in a bowl, add dissolved gelatine and allow to set. Beat egg white until just stiff then add to mixture. Fold in. Pour mixture into a dish and freeze. Remove peel and pith from orange, and slice and serve alternate layers of sorbet and orange. Decorate with a twist of orange.

Serves 2

Mrs. Wright, Rugeley Class

11

BAKED BANANAS WITH ORANGE SAUCE

2 small bananas
1½ tablespoons lemon juice
6 drops liquid sweetener

Sauce:
¼ pint unsweetened orange juice
6 drops liquid sweetener
½ level tablespoon cornflour

Peel bananas and place in dish with a little water, enough to cover the fruit. Add the liquid sweetener and lemon juice. Bake at 325°F/Gas 3 for 30 minutes.

Sauce: Blend the cornflour with a little of the orange juice to a smooth paste. Boil the rest of the orange juice and liquid sweetener, then pour on to blended cornflour. Return mixture to the saucepan and cook, stirring continuously until the sauce has thickened—about 3 minutes. Place the bananas on a serving dish and pour the sauce over them just before serving.

Serves 2

Mrs. Jean Murray, Fraserburgh Class

8

APRICOT BAKE

15-ounce tin apricots
3 ounces white breadcrumbs
1 ounce butter
1 egg
½ pint milk
1 level dessertspoon caster sugar

Drain juice from apricots. Put breadcrumbs into bowl, melt butter in pan and pour onto crumbs with apricot juice. Mix well. Put mixture into the pie-dish. Arrange apricots on top. Break egg into a bowl and gradually beat in milk. Add sugar and pour mixture round apricots. Bake at 350°F/Gas 4 for 30 to 40 minutes.

Serves 4

Mrs. B. J. Antill, Sutton Coldfield Class

49

JUBILEE SPONGE

3 eggs
4 ounces caster sugar
3 ounces self-raising flour
1 tablespoon tepid water
Jam or fruit purée to sandwich

Whisk egg whites in bowl until very stiff. Add egg yolks slowly one at a time. Stir sugar into mixture and then add tepid water. Fold in sieved flour gently with a metal spoon. Divide mixture between two greased sandwich tins and bake for ten minutes in a hot oven, 425°F/Gas 7. When baked, remove from tins and allow to cool on wire tray before sandwiching together with chosen filling.

Serves 4

Mrs. L. L. Keane, Denmead Class

49

YUM YUM CAKE

Base:
2 ounces brown sugar
3 ounces margarine
2 egg yolks
6 ounces flour
Vanilla essence

Topping:
2 egg whites
4 ounces caster sugar
1 ounce glacé cherries
1 ounce walnuts (shelled)

Base: Cream sugar and margarine together, add egg yolks and vanilla essence and fold in flour. Spread in a greased swiss roll tin.

Topping: Beat egg whites until stiff, fold in sugar, chopped cherries and nuts. Spread over base and bake in a moderate oven, 350°F/Gas 4, for 20–30 minutes.

Mrs. P. Damp, Leyland Class

94

DOOFERS

8 ounces digestive biscuits
4 ounces best margarine
2 dessertspoons drinking chocolate
1 tablespoon golden syrup
4 ounces cooking chocolate

Crush the biscuits with a rolling pin. Melt the margarine, syrup and drinking chocolate over a low heat (do not boil). Pour this mixture over the crushed biscuits. Mix together and press the mixture into a flat tin. Melt the chocolate and pour over the mixture. When cold, cut into squares.

Miss Avril Cunnington, Northampton Class

112

NUTTY TYPE LOAF

7 ounces oatmeal } **mix together and leave overnight**
$\frac{1}{2}$ pint buttermilk }
9 ounces wholemeal flour
1 teaspoon self-raising flour
1 teaspoon bicarbonate soda

Mix the flours and the bicarbonate then add to oatmeal mixture. If too dry, add a little more buttermilk. Mix well. Put all on a floured board. Shape like a round loaf and put an X on top. Sprinkle a little oatmeal on top and bake at 375°F/Gas 5 for 25 minutes.

Mrs. B. Hoarder, Portsmouth Class

73

BANANA TEA BREAD

8 ounces flour
2½ teaspoons baking powder
½ teaspoon salt
3 ounces shortening
3 ounces sugar
2 eggs (beaten)
4 ripe bananas (mashed)
4 ounces chopped nuts (mixed)

Sift together flour, baking powder and salt. Place shortening in a mixing bowl and beat until creamy; gradually add sugar, beating until light and fluffy after each addition. Add beaten eggs and beat until thick. Add flour mixture and bananas alternately, blending thoroughly after each addition. Fold in ¾ of the nuts. Turn batter into loaf tin (8 × 4 × 3 inches) which has been greased on the bottom only, and sprinkle remaining nuts on top. Bake in a moderate oven 350°F/Gas 4 for 60–70 minutes. Allow bread to cool for 20–30 minutes before turning onto rack.

Lynda Watley, Northampton Class

111

SILHOUETTE POINT VALUES FOR RECIPE INGREDIENTS

MEAT AND POULTRY 1 POINT = 25 CALORIES

		POINTS	per QUANTITY
Bacon	raw (average rasher)	**7**	1½ ounces
	fat (raw)	**7**	1 ounce
	gammon (raw)	**4**	1 ounce
Beef	(roast, lean only)	**2½**	1 ounce
	lean grilling steak (raw)	**2**	1 ounce
	fried steak	**3**	1 ounce
	stewing steak (raw)	**3**	1 ounce
	minced beef (average)	**5**	1½ ounces
	corned	**4**	1½ ounces
	canned stewed steak with onions	**30**	15½ ounce can
Beefburger	frozen	**6½**	1 ounce
Chicken	boiled (meat only)	**4½**	2 ounces
Duck	roast	**4**	1 ounce
Frankfurter	(average)	**3**	1 large
Ham	cooked (lean only)	**4**	1½ ounces
Heart	lamb's (raw)	**2**	1 ounce
Lamb	roast (lean only)	**9**	2½ ounces
	breast (lean and fat)	**6**	1 ounce
	chop (as purchased)	**14**	3 ounces
Liver	raw	**4**	2½ ounces
Luncheon Meat	(average)	**4**	1 ounce
Ox kidney	(raw)	**2**	1½ ounces
Ox tongue		**7**	2 ounces
Pork	raw (lean)	**5**	1½ ounces
	roast loin (lean and fat)	**5**	1 ounce
	belly pork (raw)	**6**	1 ounce
Sausages (averages)	beef (thick)	**7½**	1 ounce
	pork (thick)	**8½**	1 ounce
	beef sausage meat	**6**	1 ounce
	party sausage	**¾**	each
Veal	fillet (raw)	**3**	2½ ounces
	stewing (raw)	**3**	1 ounce
	cutlet fried in egg and breadcrumbs	**5**	2 ounces

FISH

		POINTS	per QUANTITY
Cod	fillets (raw)	**2**	2½ ounces
Haddock	smoked (as purchased)	**1**	1½ ounces
	" (steamed)	**1**	1 ounce

Herring	as purchased	**4**	2½ ounces
	fillets (raw)	**8**	3 ounces
Mussels	boiled	**1**	1 ounce
Plaice	fillets (raw)	**1**	1 ounce
Prawns	peeled	**2½**	2 ounces
Salmon	tinned	**3**	2 ounces
Shrimps	(peeled)	**4**	3 ounces
Skate	fillets (raw)	**1**	1 ounce
Sole	fillets (raw)	**1**	1 ounce
Trout	steamed (whole)	**3**	2½ ounces

VEGETABLES

		POINTS	per QUANTITY
Aubergine	(raw)	**1**	6 ounces
Beans	frozen green sliced	**1**	6 ounces
	haricot (raw)	**3**	1 ounce
Brussels Sprouts	(raw)	**1**	2¾ ounces
Cabbage	(raw)	**1**	3½ ounces
Carrot	(raw)	**1**	4 ounces
Cauliflower	(raw)	**1**	3½ ounces
Celery	(raw)	**1**	8 ounces
Courgette	(raw)	**1**	6 ounces
Cucumber		**1**	8 ounces
Leek	(raw)	**1**	2¾ ounces
Lettuce		**1**	8 ounces
Marrow	(raw)	**1**	6 ounces
Mushrooms	(raw)	**1**	12½ ounces
Onion	(raw)	**1**	3½ ounces
Parsnip	(raw)	**2**	3½ ounces
Peas	(frozen)	**2**	2½ ounces
Pepper	green (raw)	**1**	2¾ ounces
	red (raw)	**1**	2½ ounces
Potato	raw (as purchased)	**1**	1 ounce
	sweet (boiled)	**1**	1 ounce
Radish		**1**	6 ounces
Spinach	(frozen)	**1**	3½ ounces
Sweet Corn	(frozen)	**1**	1 ounce
Tomato	(fresh)	**1**	6 ounces
	(tinned)	**1**	4½ ounces
Watercress		**1**	6 ounces

FRUIT

		POINTS	per QUANTITY
Apple	dessert (one average)	**2**	4 ounces
	cooking (peeled and cored)	**2**	5 ounces
	,, (stewed without sugar)	**2**	5½ ounces
Apricots	canned in syrup	**1**	1 ounce
	dried (raw)	**2**	1 ounce
Banana	without skin (one average)	**2**	2½ ounces
Grapefruit	as purchased	**1**	8 ounces
Grapes	black	**1**	1½ ounces
	white	**1**	1½ ounces

Lemon	as purchased	**1**	6 ounces
	juice	**1**	12 ounces
Mandarin Oranges	canned in syrup	**1**	1½ ounces
Melon	flesh only	**1**	3½ ounces
Orange	as purchased	**1**	3 ounces
	natural juice	**1**	2½ ounces
Peaches	fresh	**1**	3 ounces
	canned in syrup	**1**	1 ounce
Pear	dessert	**2**	5 ounces
Pineapple	fresh	**1**	2 ounces
	canned in syrup	**2**	2½ ounces
Prunes	stewed without sugar	**2**	2½ ounces
Raisins		**3**	1 ounce
Rhubarb	(raw)	**1**	12 ounces
Strawberries	(fresh)	**1**	3 ounces
Sultanas		**3**	1 ounce

NUTS

		POINTS per	QUANTITY
Almonds	shelled	**7**	1 ounce
Chestnuts	without shell	**2**	1 ounce
Walnuts	shelled	**6**	1 ounce
Mixed Nuts	shelled (average)	**6**	1 ounce

FATS AND DAIRY PRODUCE

		POINTS per	QUANTITY
Butter		**9**	1 ounce
Buttermilk		**4½**	½ pint
Cheese	Cheddar	**7**	1½ ounces
	Danish Blue	**4**	1 ounce
	Gruyère	**8**	1½ ounces
	Parmesan	**3**	¾ ounce
	Cream cheese (depending on fat content)	**6–10**	1 ounce
	Cottage cheese	**3**	2½ ounces
Cream	single	**5**	2 ounces
	double	**8**	1½ ounces
	sour cream	**4½**	2 ounces
Dream Topping	whipped	**2**	1½ fluid ounces
Egg	standard	**3½**	1 ounce
Evaporated Milk	tinned	**2**	1 fluid ounce
Lard		**10½**	1 ounce
Margarine		**9**	1 ounce
Milk	silver or red top	**15**	pint
	gold top	**19½**	pint
Oil	corn oil	**10½**	1 ounce
	olive oil	**10½**	1 ounce
Suet		**10½**	1 ounce
Yogurt	natural (unsweetened)	**3**	5 ounces

CEREALS AND STARCHES

		POINTS	per QUANTITY
Arrowroot		**4**	1 ounce
Biscuits	digestive	**5½**	1 ounce
	semi-sweet (mixed)	**5**	1 ounce
	sweet (mixed)	**6½**	1 ounce
Bread	white or brown	**4**	1½ ounces
	fresh breadcrumbs	**4**	1½ ounces
Cornflour		**4**	1 ounce
Custard Powder		**4**	1 ounce
Flour		**4**	1 ounce
Noodles	raw	**4**	1 ounce
	boiled	**2**	1½ ounces
Oatmeal	raw	**4½**	1 ounce
Puff Pastry	frozen	**5**	1 ounce
Ravioli	canned	**2**	1½ ounces
Rice	raw	**4**	1 ounce
	boiled	**4**	3 ounces
Spaghetti	raw	**4**	1 ounce
	boiled	**4**	3 ounces

SUGARY FOODS

		POINTS	per QUANTITY
Angelica		**3½**	1 ounce
Chocolate	plain	**6**	1 ounce
Glacé Apricots		**2**	1 ounce
Cherries		**3**	1 ounce
Golden Syrup		**5**	1½ ounces
Honey		**5**	1½ ounces
Ice Cream	plain	**4½**	2 ounces
	Cornish	**5½**	2 ounces
Jam		**3**	1 ounce
Jelly	packet (sweetened)	**3**	1 ounce
	gelatine	**4**	1½ ounces
Lemon Curd		**3½**	1 ounce
Stem Ginger		**3½**	1 ounce
Sugar	white or brown (granulated or caster)	**4½**	1 ounce
Treacle	black	**3**	1 ounce

DRINKS

		POINTS	per QUANTITY
Ale	light	**1**	3 fluid ounces
Brandy		**5**	2 fluid ounces
Cider	dry	**1**	2½ fluid ounces
Cocoa Powder		**2½**	½ ounce
Curaçao		**3**	liqueur measure
Drinking Chocolate		**2½**	½ ounce
Ginger Ale	dry	**2**	5 fluid ounces
Ginger Beer		**1**	2 fluid ounces
Lemon Barley		**2**	1½ fluid ounces
Lime Juice Cordial		**2**	1½ fluid ounces
Orange Squash	undiluted	**1½**	1 fluid ounce
Sherry	medium sweet	**3**	2 fluid ounces
Wine	dry white (average)	**2**	2½ fluid ounces
	dry red (average)	**2**	2½ fluid ounces

SAUCES, PICKLES AND SOUP

		POINTS	per QUANTITY
Brown Sauce		**1**	1 ounce
Curry Powder		**1½**	½ ounce
Horseradish Sauce		**½**	3 tablespoons
Mayonnaise		**4½**	1 ounce
Mushroom Soup	(1 packet × 1 pint)	**8**	packet
Olives	stuffed	**1**	3
Oxtail Soup	(1 packet × 1 pint)	**6½**	packet
Sweet Pickles		**3**	2 ounces
Tomato Juice		**1**	4 ounces
Tomato Ketchup		**1**	1 ounce
Tomato Purée		**1**	2 tablespoons
Condensed Soup	1 can × 10½ ounces average	**9**	

FREE LIST

Because of the small quantities in which they are used in the recipes, the following ingredients have negligible Point Value:

Condiments – salt, peppers, vinegars, Worcestershire sauce
Herbs
Spices
Meat and Yeast Extracts
Clear Stocks
Flavouring Essences
No-Calorie Sweetening Agents (e.g. Saccharine)

SILHOUETTE AREA MANAGERS UK & EIRE

ABERDEEN	Iris Goodall 159 Bon Accord Street, Aberdeen Telephone Aberdeen 27506
BERKS., BUCKS. AND OXFORD	Jean Slatter 7 Niagara Road, Henley-on-Thames, RG9 1EB Telephone Henley 4037
CHESHIRE AND SOUTH LANCS.	Valerie Bell 5 Maltmans Road, Lymm, Cheshire Telephone Lymm 2520
DERBY, NOTTS., STAFFS., AND SALOP	Beryl Davies Rose Hill, Stoney Lane, Endon, Stoke-on-Trent, ST9 9EX Telephone 503182
DUNDEE AND PERTH	Valerie Leslie 8d Gleneagles Court, Ardler, Dundee Telephone Dundee 89538
DURHAM AND NORTHUMBERLAND	Helen Dobbie, 39 Woodburn Drive, Whitley Bay, Northumberland Telephone Whitley Bay 25648
EAST AND CENTRAL YORKSHIRE	Doris Peirson 27 Pullan Drive, Bradford, BD2 3RW Telephone Bradford 638653
EAST DORSET	Norma Small 7 Stanfield Road, Ferndown, Dorset Telephone Ferndown 3128
EDINBURGH	Nancy Fraser 38 Northfield Crescent, Edinburgh 8 Telephone 661 2182
EIRE	Evelyn Murphy 17 Rose Park, Kill Avenue, Dunlaoghaire, Co. Dublin Telephone Dublin 807968
GLASGOW EAST	Marie McPhail 48 Golf Drive, Glasgow, G15 6TA Telephone 944 4463
GLASGOW NORTH	Ann Andrew 5 Menzies Drive, Fintry, Glasgow, G63 0YG Telephone Fintry 388
GLASGOW SOUTH	Ruby Allison 5 Westburn Avenue, Cambuslang, Glasgow Telephone 641 1664

HAMPSHIRE, I.O.W.	Jean Hanley 96 Regents Park Road, Southampton Telephone Southampton 57388 from 9–5 and Southampton 78563 after 6
KENT AND WEST SUSSEX	Patricia Bradford 2 Enfield Road, Deal, Kent Telephone Deal 5175
LANCS. AND WESTMORLAND	Marion Murphy Tara, Kingsdown Crescent, Wigan, Lancs.
LINCOLN AND WEST YORKSHIRE	Vilma Hazelhurst Carl-Haze, Royston Road, Shafton, Yorks. Telephone Cudworth 585
MID-WEST	Dora Aspin 59 Woodhill Road, Portishead, Somerset, BS20 9EY Telephone Portishead 3412
NORFOLK, SUFFOLK AND ESSEX	Margaret Keelde Grays, 56 Highfields Road, Witham, Essex Telephone Witham 2037
NORTHANTS., LEICS., CAMBS., HUNTINGDON, RUTLAND, BEDS.	Madge Gosling 79 Overstone Road, Moulton, Northants. Telephone Northampton 43962
NORTH-EAST AND SOUTH LONDON	Patricia Harper 1 Thames Meadows, Hurst Park, West Molesey, KT8 9TQ Telephone 01 979 9497
NORTH LONDON AND HERTS.	Freda Vincent 48 Brandles Road, Letchworth, Herts., SG6 2JB Telephone 981 932 6908
NORTH WALES	Joan Irving 12 Clayton Drive, Prestatyn, Flints. Telephone Prestatyn 4132
NORTH-WEST LONDON, BUCKS., AND HERTS.	Daphne Badrock 2a Dickinson Square, Croxley Green, Herts, WO3 3EZ Telephone Rickmansworth 75518
SOUTH WALES	Sheila Carter 61 Llandyry, Felinfoel, Llanelli, Carmarthen
SOUTH-WEST	Jennifer Sampson 24 Hill Close, Pennsylvania, Exeter, Devon Telephone Exeter 76775
SURREY AND SUSSEX	Rosalie Johns 121 Cabell Road, Park Barn, Guildford, Surrey Telephone Guildford 77846
WARWICKSHIRE	Maureen Boddington 12 Redacre Road, Boldmere, Sutton Coldfield, Warwickshire Telephone 021 354 3592
WIRRAL, CHESHIRE	Audrey Spencer 15 Sandrock Road, Marford, Nr. Wrexham, Denbighs.

INDEX

SILHOUETTE RECIPES

SWEETS

VEGETABLES AND SALADS